Challenges and Choices for Patient, Carer and Professional at the End of Life

T0386482

Living with Uncertainty gives a broad perspective on the complexities and challenges of the practice of end-of-life care, as well as the perceived benefits and limitations of medical intervention.

Drawn from research and clinical and pastoral experience, the book examines the feelings associated with the end of life, highlighting the demands that people are faced with and their consequences. It moves into the difficult area of people who feel defeated by their illness and can or want to live no longer, as well as the family, caregivers and professionals who surround them. These perspectives have been built upon around a hundred narratives of lived experience, combined with the wider clinical and practical range of voices. A topical post-script *Lessons from Covid-19* captures the choices and challenges on a personal, professional and systemic level which the pandemic acutely revealed with a multiplicity of examples.

This will be essential reading for students and professionals in palliative and end-of-life care. Families and friends will also benefit from this book as they try to come to terms with the delicate but universal issues of death and dying.

Catherine Proot holds an MSc in psychology and education from Ghent University, Belgium, a Postgraduate Diploma in counselling and a PhD from the UEA in Norwich, UK. A psychotherapist and clinical supervisor, she has specialised in palliative and bereavement care since 2005 in the UK and Belgium. She works in private practice in Brussels.

The **Very Revd Michael Yorke** (1939–2019) was a Cambridge graduate in law and theology. An Anglican Priest, he worked principally in and through four cathedrals. He was for 18 years a Samaritan, three of them as National Chairman, and was Vice Chairman to the Norfolk Hospice near Kings Lynn, UK.

Challenges and Choices for Patient, Carer and Professional at the End of Life

Living with Uncertainty

Catherine Proot and
Michael Yorke

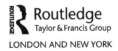
Routledge
Taylor & Francis Group

LONDON AND NEW YORK

First published 2021
by Routledge
2 Park Square, Milton Park, Abingdon, Oxon OX14 4RN

and by Routledge
52 Vanderbilt Avenue, New York, NY 10017

Routledge is an imprint of the Taylor & Francis Group, an informa business

British Library Cataloguing-in-Publication Data
A catalogue record for this book is available from the British Library

Library of Congress Cataloging-in-Publication Data
A catalog record has been requested for this book

ISBN: 978-0-367-54447-8 (hbk)
ISBN: 978-0-367-54446-1 (pbk)
ISBN: 978-1-003-08934-6 (ebk)

Typeset in Sabon
by Apex CoVantage, LLC

Contents

Foreword

I write this foreword in extraordinary times. The global COVID-19 pandemic has led us to re-evaluate and reflect on the way in which we lead our lives and what the future holds for us as people, citizens and indeed, health care professionals. It has also brought the reality of death and dying to the fore and, in many ways, addresses the scope of this book, living with uncertainty. In addition to the global shock to our daily lives, enforced isolation, separation from family and friends, the risk of traumatic and sudden death, inability to say goodbye to loved ones, attend funerals and share the essential death and grief rituals which aid our transition to loss will leave an indelible imprint on society and, perhaps, remind us of the fragility of our human existence.

At the same time, these challenges have opened a door to positive elements for our future living as community; stronger engagement, a sense of deeper listening and respect for the care given and received by others and for self. As Catherine Proot and the late Michael Yorke present in their second evocative book, these elements involve choice and being able to live well with the choices made, however difficult that may be.

What is most interesting about this book is that it does not attempt to postulate new theory but rather addresses questions that we, in palliative and end-of-life care, have discussed across many years. What is a good death? What is quality of life? How do we determine our professional or clinical identity? The authors take us on a thoughtful and judicious pathway through complex arguments and situate those within the voice of practitioners who live those questions every day of their working lives. And of course, they address the complex phenomena of right to live and right to die. As a palliative care nurse, writing from the Republic of Ireland where euthanasia and assisted dying are rare in discourse but working in Switzerland where assisted dying is part of the clinical vernacular, I find myself drawn in to the varied perspectives exposed by those interviewed in the book. I sense their dilemma, and the flow between the author's writing and the words of the respondents enable a meaningful reflection on how their choices impact on me as a professional and an academic. And so, for the reader, I hope that this book will enable you to make sense of the unique contribution you make to the individual experience of death and dying.

A phrase which echoes through this book is the 'twilight of life'. Twilight defines the end of the day, the movement from light to dark, a time of rest and quiet. Standing in the twilight, the world seems to change in colour and tone. Things become fuzzy. Clinicians often have to make their most profound decisions and choices in a fuzzy and ever-changing landscape. The honest stories presented here attest to the 'fuzziness' of death and dying and its personal and professional impact on us, sometimes positive, sometimes not. Ultimately, this book is about how we help patients and families to make the right choices in their twilight. In her book *The Choice*, Dr Edith Eger argues that you cannot change what happened in the past but you can choose what happens now. Helping people to make the right choice takes courage and commitment. This book will help you to understand why that is so important at this challenging time as we reframe our understanding of end of life.

Philip Larkin
Kristian Gerhard Jebsen Chair of Palliative Care Nursing
University of Lausanne, Switzerland

Preface

This book builds on our previously published work called *Life to Be Lived* (Proot & Yorke, 2014). It was a study of the challenges and choices for patients and caregivers in life-threatening illnesses. This book is about how people approach death, prepare for and endure the process of dying as a destiny which awaits all living creatures, including us human beings. It is the one certainty in life. This volume extends that of our first book into the difficult area of people who feel defeated by their illness and can or want to live no longer and the people around them: family, caregivers and professionals.

We have not found it an easy book to write, for the experience of death is widely feared, almost universally queried as to its nature and what is to follow, if anything. The impact of such questions has not allowed us to be immune from challenging reactions. Some of the ideas we share with you were considered, sometimes in depth, in the first book; but many of the issues relating to dying raise different ethical and moral challenges and controversy. Within this huge picture, we will consider the role of medicine in life saving and life ending, for instance, when is a life support machine to be turned off or not. We discuss euthanasia and abortion as well as the preserving of life regardless of the consequences in the future for the patient.

We do not set out to expound new attitudes and concepts. We seek to interpret those that are current and how they affect the people of today. As the discoveries, skills and medicine advance, we believe that contemporary ethics should be under constant review. A case can be considered with euthanasia as the subject. There is plenty of disagreement and constructive and strong feelings to prove the point.

This book is not specifically about euthanasia, but we are writing against a background of increasing curiosity and indeed specific legislation in the Low Countries allowing life-shortening interventions. This is why a number of our stories refer to this reality and how people respond to it. This does not indicate an approval of these practices, but they are highly relevant to the debates about end-of-life care in our Western society.

We have thought it interesting to contribute to these debates by collecting stories and experiences of people involved in care at the end of life both in the UK, where euthanasia and physician-assisted dying are illegal, and in the Low Countries, where there is a legislation allowing patients to request euthanasia and it to be permitted and carried out under certain and specific conditions. We have interviewed consultants in oncology and palliative care, GPs, nurses, psychologists, supervisors, spiritual carers and volunteers working in a range of settings such as hospice, community, hospital and university, on both sides of the Channel. For all information in this book, we rely on the stories told to us by our informants, which, using narrative (Riessman, 2002, 1993) and interpretative phenomenological analysis (Shaw, 2001; Smith, Flowers, & Larkin, 2009), we have ordered and sorted in a way in which the collected information made sense and could lead our readers into a deeper understanding of the twilight of life.

Echoing the voice of people who have direct experience, including those who have dealt with patients who choose for or against euthanasia, their families and caregivers, and professionals who have been involved in deliberating and performing the act, the book provides engaging and relevant examples and quotes to illustrate the complexity of the issues involved. Our approach is a pastoral one, looking at how these different realities impact people's experiences, hopes and fears towards the end of life. Addressing the topic from the perspectives of patient/caregiver and of volunteer/professional reminds the reader at the outset of the impact of so-called autonomous decisions that they are communal, relational in their impact and not limited to the individual who makes the decision.

The European Association of Palliative Care wishes for studies of attitudes to, and experiences about euthanasia and physician-assisted suicide among professionals, patients and the wider public to inform the debate (Radbruch et al., 2016, p. 16). We hope that this book may contribute to this and that whoever reads it may feel valued and affirmed in their experience, whatever that may be, and look to their death with steady endurance, confidence and thanksgiving.

We have used direct quotations from clinicians and others who have been generous in the time they have given us. We have used their wisdom and experience to clarify these contemporary attitudes and to assist us in developing our own views. The aim is to help our readers to think again as to where they stand in the important issues of today. As a pair of writers, we have not always agreed on a line of thought and expect the same may happen amongst our readership. We hope that the many voices in the stories and the wealth of information and experience they provide can inform each individual to recognise their own and reach a judgement for their future. As in *Life to Be Lived*, we have divided the text into chapters and sections, and each can stand on its own, although they are all a part of a complex whole.

The book is written for volunteers and multidisciplinary professionals training in palliative medicine and end-of-life care, and we have included some questions after each chapter to trigger their thinking and reflection.

We hope it will also assist the broader public, particularly patients with a life-limiting illness and their caregivers and families who wish to reflect on their responses to the situation they are in. We have been particularly cautious about protecting the anonymity of our informants and the subjects of their stories, and thus all who have personally helped us are given a pseudonym in the text.

We hope that this book will contribute to a better understanding of and respect for the motivations and attitudes behind patients' wishes and focus towards the end of life – be it to end their life deliberately or choose not to do so – and thus to improve the capacity to offer appropriate holistic care and psychosocial and spiritual support in the twilight of life. We trust that people involved in any way in palliative and end-of-life care will find this book a repository of valuable resources as they journey towards the inevitability of their own dying and that of their patients and clients. Honouring the variety of ways to live one's dying and that everyone's dying is unique, we hope you, our readers, will see or hear messages of assistance and clarification for your own experience.

References

Proot, C. & Yorke, M., 2014. *Life to Be Lived: Challenges and Choices for Patients and Carers in Life-threatening Illnesses.* Oxford: Oxford University Press.

Radbruch, L., Leget, C., Bahr, P., Muller-Busch, C., Ellershaw, J., De Conno, F. & Vanden Berghe, P., 2016. Euthanasia and Physician-Assisted Suicide: A White Paper from the European Association for Palliative Care. *Palliative Medicine*, Volume 30 (2), pp. 104–116.

Riessman, C., 1993. *Narrative Analysis.* London: Sage.

Riessman, C., 2002. Narrative Analysis. In: A. M. Huberman & M. R. Miles, eds., *The Qualitative Researcher's Companion.* London: Sage.

Shaw, R., 2001. Why Use Interpretative Phenomenological Analysis in Health Psychology? *Health Psychology Update*, Volume 10, pp. 48–52.

Smith, J., Flowers, P. & Larkin, M., 2009. *Interpretative Phenomenological Analysis: Theory, Method and Research.* London: Sage.

Acknowledgements

We are immensely grateful to the many who have contributed directly or indirectly towards this project. Among them we record our thanks to the interviewees who gave at least three hours of their time and showed a willingness to be honest and critical about their own methods, strengths and feelings; to all the people who have made available their insight and experience; and to those who have checked the text, provided for our comfort and encouraged us to continue when the going became tough. Among them we would like to mention by name:

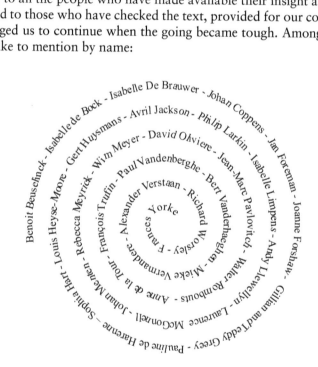

With a mixture of joy and reflection we remember Michael Yorke, who died before seeing this volume in print. His motivation and contribution to completing the book have been invaluable even if sometimes he has felt a strong irony in the timing.

Introduction

Many of us who drive a vehicle will recognise the increased difficulty in judging speed, distance or space as daylight recedes and twilight begins. The added difficulty of making judgements and having blunted awareness can increase our liability to make mistakes or become confused in interpreting what is ahead of us – therefore, accidents are more likely to occur. Such testing has application to life in general. If drivers have difficulties in seeing their way to drive well in the twilight, it is all the more important for those who are disadvantaged in some way through health, circumstance or background to be given help in steering through the twilight of their life successfully. Sadly, this is not always the case, which therefore leads to increased sense of disadvantage, failure and pointlessness and an increase in the number of suicides.

Medical intervention generally reaches an individual person because they become ill or suffer an accident or neglect. Objectively it can be a quite minor issue, but for the person involved it may be anything but minor. Such experiences span a wide range of events. It may be the use of drugs such as paracetamol to ease pain, a sedative to help sleep or some physical action to alleviate a toothache or acute muscle pain. Medical involvement in a person's life or even their death may be the other end of the spectrum, but the motive and the appropriate skill are relevant to all. Like life itself, medicine is a patchwork quilt of good things and bad. We were told that the best drug for a sick person is the doctor's time. However, time is money, and good medical care, wherever it takes place, is very expensive, so it is a vital political as well as a social challenge to us all.

The medical picture is changing from absolute dependence on the skill and experience of the doctor to scientific criteria which are sensitive to the cost of responsibility and liability to economic pressures. Good care for the very ill can be provided in the agencies through loving attention and presence, which help the patient to look positively at their position. This can be difficult if the diagnosis is threatening to life and is given without sensitivity and awareness of the consequences. We need as much help as we can get as we all face this universal reality of dying: that great event which none of us can avoid even if we wish to ignore it. There should be a sense of community in which the patient is included and given a status, especially when they feel weak, depressed or anxious about the future. They should be helped to value the here and now and to recognise what they have achieved in earlier life. The consequential wholeness given by such an approach can help the patient to make choices about what should happen in the future.

We are aware of the occasional tension between medically orientated practice and palliative care as we see it, i.e. total care of body, mind, spirit and social relationships. We seek to indicate the strengths of scientific and clinical medicine and of palliative and end-of-life care while following the concerns and attitudes of those who are at the receiving end of them and draw out some of the differences in approach and priorities and to comment on them. As in our previous book, *Life to Be Lived* (2014), the focus is on the feelings and mindsets of patients who approach their dying and those immediately involved as family, friends, caregivers and the medical, nursing and other professionals. As we understand more about what lies before us, it is our hope that we will contribute some learning which could be important to all of us at some unknown future date.

Death is normal. It is inevitable in all living creatures. However, it may be 'abnormal' in how it occurs. There is always some sort of suffering for the person concerned, unless maybe when death is instantaneous, in which case the shock, suffering and concerns for the people left behind can be close to unbearable. The suffering may be conscious or unconscious; it can even be beyond our control, for instance in the struggling for breath. On the other hand, for the dying person and around the deathbed there may be a sense of peace or relief, whether it is expressed or not.

The process of even 'normal' death can be disturbing and can cause distress, especially when we are witnessing it for the first time or when we have been party to a difficult or traumatic death in the past. In some families, there can be a growing pressure on professional caregivers to force things. They wonder, 'What is the meaning of this suffering? Why can't the doctor do something?' This can be difficult for the medical staff when they see, based on their experience and professional expertise, that this specific dying process is going smoothly in their view, and there is no suffering which requires intervention. They have to recognise that for the family it is not always easy to watch someone dying and find ways to support them at this difficult time.

Dying is the normal final part of our life, and it is crucially important. Even if there are no big problems with pain or other symptoms, there is still that process of being able to let go of the family and one's surroundings and saying goodbye. A palliative care physician told us:

> I remember seeing a woman who had died. I had to go and certify that she was dead. The curtains were drawn around her, and the soft morning light coming through from the windows was beautiful. It felt incredibly peaceful. Sometimes it doesn't feel like that, but with her I thought, 'Yes, something good has happened here'.

Just like this physician, we can have an experience of fulfilment when we are witnessing the final part of someone's life. There seems to be something unique or different about preparing for the end of a life. We all have heard or read of stories about how people close to death seem to be at a border between two worlds, conscious of both sides of the doorway, as it were (Moody, 1975, 2001; Giacino & White, 2005; McCullagh, 2004). They are aware of their family sitting with them but also of something more, another dimension and its inhabitants. Some people may be psychotic or hallucinating near death, but many are not. They may just be experiencing another reality. Some speak about being welcomed to that farther shore, as many hope they will be. What could be more important than that fullness of hope!

These are question marks, and there can be no certainties. However, we all hold beliefs, expectations and attitudes about death and dying which will impact our experiences. We have chosen in the first part of the book to look more closely at some of these beliefs and attitudes that have been revealed by the interviewees and our personal experience. We consider people's fears, hopes, beliefs and assumptions about death and dying and describe real-life experiences of how people have coped with their end-of-life journey, their feelings and ordeals and the challenges of loss, trauma, pain and suffering.

The second part of the book focuses on medicine and care in the twilight of life. When people are ageing and nearing the end of their life, their encounters with the medical and nursing professions increase considerably. For some it is a sudden dip into new – and often foreign – territory with its codes and ethics they do not yet understand. Others gradually become more involved, yet they too feel helpless, and when the end draws near, they realise they are not really prepared.

Can anything really prepare us for this inevitable mystery? It will probably be each and everyone's own personal journey, but in line with the purpose of this book, we thought it useful in the second part to have a closer look at what medicine and care at the twilight of life can look like, if only to clear out some fantasies, beliefs and misconceptions that might stand in the way of making the most of that precious time. In a world where, medically, one can be kept alive or put to sleep, the issues of 'quality of life' and 'quality of death' will be considered in some depth. A post-script completes our reflection with lessons learnt from Covid-19.

As we examine the moral, technical and ethical challenges of medical intervention, the move to Belgium of one of the writers has created the opportunity to describe the impact of the law on euthanasia and assisted dying in the Low Countries, 15 years on, and compare that with the heated debate on the subject in the UK. We further consider the difficult decisions and end-of-life conversations doctors are facing and the impact of advance directives and advance care planning. As both of us have been closely involved with hospices, one clinically and the other managerially and structurally, we discuss in a final chapter what the palliative approach and person-centred care have to offer in the twilight of life.

In order to clarify and demonstrate the issues at stake as the end of life approaches, we will recount stories given to us by those whom we have interviewed or which arise from our own clinical experience. As a result, some are amusing, some deeply saddening – but they all testify to some aspect of human life towards the end of life. This is not a theoretical or philosophical book; it is about life with all the delights and failures. It is, we hope, eminently practical and helpful to those who turn to it, wherever they may stand at that particular time.

As we write this book, we are aware that most of us will grow to some degree of old age. If someone is snatched from life at an early age, as a child or young person, most of us will feel particularly saddened with the feeling that a young person has been cheated of life. We assume that we have the right to expect a number of years in which we will be able to work and have a family and a reasonably happy and contented later life. Most importantly, the sense that we have contributed something to the world will figure strongly in our sense of achievement. The twilight of life can be lovely or contain a big sense of loss of opportunity. For all of us, the reality of death can provoke new feelings and fears associated with daily life.

There are no clear indicators about what the future will be. Death is the great unknown. We have lots of different ways of approaching mystery. One is perhaps through philosophy, one is through science, one is through religion . . . but we need always to be very careful, when we approach mystery, never to assume that because we are looking through rose-tinted lenses the entire world is rosy. We are influenced by our lens. To be a good professional one needs to look at the world through our lens and be able to use our lens, but one will be a better doctor or a better nurse to recognise their limitation and perhaps the value of other lenses too. We hope our approach and openness will assist our readers in finding what they search for even in the twilight.

References

Giacino, J. & White, J., 2005. The Vegetative and Minimally Conscious States: Current Knowledge and Remaining Questions. *The Journal of Head Trauma and Rehabilitation*, Volume 20, pp. 30–50.

McCullagh, P., 2004. *Conscious in a Vegetative State? A Critique of the PVS Concept*. Dordrecht: Kluwer Academic Publishers.

Moody, R. J., 1975, 2001. *Life after Life: The Investigation of a Phenomenon – Survival of Bodily Death*. New York: HarperCollins Publishers.

Proot, C. & Yorke, M., 2014. *Life to Be Lived: Challenges and Choices for Patients and Carers in Life-threatening Illnesses*. Oxford: Oxford University Press.

Part I

The dying person and their loved ones

Chapter 1

Attitudes to death and dying

Although set within inevitability and universality in creation, death is unique to each person or creature involved. Within the uniqueness and universality of death and dying, there is a great unknown, and this occurs equally among those who look to no future beyond death and among those who have a faith that death is not a permanent ending but a door to something new or different. Even with people who have been distressed during their final illness, it is important to recognise that we have little idea what is going on inside their hearts and heads when they are close to death, even when seemingly unconscious. We might imagine that they are just asleep, but there may be a lot more happening than we realise. It is well known that people who appear to be unconscious seem able to retain the capacity of hearing, even when they cannot respond (Giacino & White, 2005; McCullagh, 2004).

Some people seem to choose their moment of dying just when their loved one who has been sitting with them for days goes out of the room to get a cup of tea, as if wishing not to distress the person accompanying them. It may be a form of courtesy or concern for their loved one or something else. On the other hand, it may be the desperate wish of their family for them to stay here on earth that holds patients back from dying. Perhaps they can only complete their journey alone. Others who were deeply unconscious suddenly wake up, speaking with their family as if to say goodbye, and then lapse back into a coma only to die an hour or two later. Other mentally lucid dying people happily report seeing family members who have died or even angels. Life does not end until the last breath, and that can be difficult to identify. So who are we to decide from our external and hence limited point of view what a good death is and when it is completed?!

We like to think that, when offered the chance, people may well die as they lived. Why would someone who has always been quick to shout and kick suddenly become like a lamb, quiet and submissive, at the time of death? It seems much more likely that people's responses to the unknown and how they have learnt to deal with it all through their life will be repeated and exacerbated when facing the great unknown in death. Thus, for some, the excitement of finding something new can be real, and therefore they may well look on death as yet another exciting experience. As one old lady known to us said, "Death is the last great adventure!"

No one really knows what is on the other side of that door. Beliefs about what happens after we die are based on personal conjectures, which stem from our own curiosity and/or from transmission of a view of death and dying within our society, within our family and peers and within our community of faith and religion. They are not based on certain, experienced knowledge. Death arouses strong feelings among most people. It is part of the order of things, and sensitivity must be the watchword for all who care for the dying and the dead. We may share our creation with them, and, like them, we will one day have our turn to leave the world we know, and experience death and that world we do not yet know.

What makes a good death?

As we attempt to describe the human experience of death and dying, we want to examine what people consider to be a good death. All of us carry fantasies of how we would like to die – for instance at home, with family, listening to music, overlooking the garden, or slipping away, leaving us unaware that it happens. We also may hold fears around the validity of our hopes, for instance whether the children will be able to look after us at the end of our lives. Yet what we experience at our death may be very different from any expectation and hopes we may hold. We will never know until the time comes.

Beliefs about death and dying will be unique to each person, but there could be some recurring or striking features. We thought it worthwhile to ask our interviewees – as they come into contact with death on a regular basis with many different people and families – what they think. Their views about what they have experienced as 'a good death' are wide ranging. Analysing their responses, some qualities come to the fore, which we illustrate with stories they have told us.

In our consideration of the dying experience and the death which follows, we want to clarify that what we describe are some of the beliefs and expectations people carry, which have an impact on how they feel and behave at the twilight of life. At no point is it our purpose to define what a good death is, because despite the increasing number of tools measuring quality of life,[1] this is indescribable in our present state of knowledge and perception. That will come when the event occurs to each of us. Perhaps we would say, "Too late!"

Everyone has to die their own death, even me

A chaplain who has been working for 25 years in a major university hospital feels very strongly that nobody can know what makes 'a good death' and coined this telling statement: "Everybody has to die on their own; everybody has to die their own death".

In palliative care settings like hospices, hospitals or nursing homes, people sometimes want to have frameworks they can use for ensuring 'a good death' in which there is peace and support. While these frameworks can be very helpful, it can also happen that patients are forced to die according to such a framework, and this does not always feel right. People in the UK, for instance, have felt ill-treated by the Liverpool Care Pathway, which is now no longer in use. It was a procedure that a number of hospitals applied during what was expected to be the last hours of a patient's life. It encouraged the staff to check regularly on the needs of the dying person and their family, ensuring that they were comfortable physically, emotionally, psychologically and spiritually, while being realistic about their capacity at the time (Seymour & Clark, 2018). Unfortunately, patients and families did not always understand the purpose of some of the measures and why they were put into place. Their concern and anxiety for their loved one soared, for instance, when the dying person was not given a drink they had asked for. They were not told – or did not understand – that the patient might not be able to swallow properly and that fluid would end up in their lungs, causing greater distress.

Communication is a big issue in end-of-life care, and we will discuss this later in depth, but as one of our informants told us, one can propose or explain or show people a way to go about coping with death and dying which, based on our experience, might be 'good'. However, ultimately, people have to die their own death, so the framework may turn out to have been inappropriate. If they want to die in denial, they have the right to do so. If they want to die at home, they have the right to die at home. If they want to remain conscious till the end, even at the cost of huge pain, they have the right to that choice. The following story, told by a GP, exemplifies how a person can die their own death:

> I was caring for a young man, we'll call him Peter, whom I had known for many years. A paramedic in his early forties, Peter had four children aged 12 to 16 when he was diagnosed with stomach cancer. Having spent three weeks in hospital, he was still in a lot of pain and vomiting when he went home. We started subcutaneous drugs, which helped with vomiting quite rapidly and he was feeling relatively better for a few weeks, although he was frail and tired.
>
> In the weeks that followed, we began to talk about the fact that death could come quite soon. Peter had very young children and felt responsible for them. It was difficult for this gentleman to die. Not really for himself, but because he would be leaving behind his young family, while they still had to study for many years. His spouse had been a housewife, so financial issues and the responsibility for the children was a big problem.

After a few weeks, things deteriorated. Peter was really tired, and vomiting became worse as it restarted. We changed the drugs a bit, but it didn't work, and we decided on sedation. I worked together with a really good nurse in the village. Technically, it went well. We needed a lot of drugs and had to change the syringe driver quite frequently. It was a difficult task for the nurse, and we shared the responsibility; sometimes she would visit to change the syringe driver, other times I would.

What was so beautiful was that it was summertime, and when I visited the family, they were always in the garden. Sometimes I visited quite late after I had completed my consultations, and then I might stay and sit with them, drinking a beer. Peter did not want a hospital bed. He wanted to die on the sofa where he had been sitting for many weeks. It was not that easy for the nurse to care for him on the sofa, but she accepted it, and when we started sedation, he lay down on the sofa. After a day or so, he woke up for a few minutes only.

Peter's children were in the Boy Scouts, and for the two or three days that the sedation lasted they took their sleeping bags and their mattresses and put them on the living room floor, and they slept around him. It felt so natural, while it was particularly sad because Peter was so young and he would soon die. It was the way the family coped, even the young children, which was beautiful. It was so balanced, it helped the nurse and myself a lot. It felt like a privilege for us to be part of it.

After Peter died, I recall his wife saying "Now you are part of the family". It is a bit exaggerated, because you are not part of the family; you remain a GP doing your work. However, it is like the biggest compliment I could receive. If you can do things like that with a family, your relationship with them is never the same afterwards. It was a gift in my professional and my personal life to experience that. My relationship with the family changed as their GP.

This is the story of a very personal death, even to the detail of wanting to die on the sofa, which was not comfortable for the patient, for the nurse, nor for anybody in fact. For this family, the way it went was the way they wanted it to go. To be able to die amidst his family was made possible for Peter through the commitment of the GP and the nurse, but if you can do it like that, it contributes to what we might term 'a good death' for that family. So much so that Peter's spouse would say to the GP afterwards, "You are part of the family now!"

Shared humanity

What made Peter's and other deaths particularly good for this GP was that there had been a kind of exchange of feelings. It was not only the doctor or the nurse caring for Peter and his family, it was also the other way around:

the family cared for the GP and the nurse; they found a way that felt appropriate for everyone.

This reminds us of another story about Veronica.[2] When death drew near and Veronica became housebound, Joanne, her therapist, who had been journeying with her for more than three years, visited Veronica in her home as 'a companion on the journey'. As a result, there would be no further professional fee. Joanne wrote about her experience towards the end of Veronica's life:

> During the last week of her life I saw Veronica once, but each day I supported her husband and her friend as they nursed her with Macmillan nurses. I remember collecting the first prescription of morphine, being part of the 'case conference' with the GP in her home and sitting by her an hour or two after she died, saying my goodbyes.
>
> At her funeral, I read a story she wrote. I think of her every year at the anniversary. I remember the sand tray[3] and always the little black figure in the corner of the tray – I guess it represented her fear. Veronica would bring a summer iris, rolled up tight, and we would put it in water and during the session it would open out.

Peter's GP and Veronica's therapist became involved with their terminally ill client's family and friends towards the end and shared their humanity with them. It seemed a natural move, as if from journeying deeply with a dying patient, they became personally involved and felt a sense of responsibility to support the client's nearest and dearest in a way the patient would have wanted them to. Sharing this crucial time with the family changed their relationship. Joanne has kept in touch with Veronica's husband for many years after her death, albeit from afar.

When a patient thinks about requesting euthanasia, they may not always be abreast of what this request involves for the doctor they are talking to about it. The following story puts this in perspective.

> Phil, a respected local figure named 'their hero' by his followers in political and unionist circles, was very sick and told his GP: "I don't want to live my life until it begins to peter out. When it is getting very tough, I would like you to perform euthanasia". This GP had personal problems with this practice and was not ready to perform euthanasia. He consulted a colleague who was a palliative care physician, and they discussed the conflict the GP found himself in: He did not want to abandon his patient and could hear Phil's request, yet he had moral and personal issues at the thought of causing someone's death, let alone his patient's.
>
> What was really beautiful about Phil's situation was that his family understood very well the personal feelings of their GP, who had been their GP for many years. They respected his feelings and knew how difficult it was for him.

> After several weeks, the GP said to the palliative care physician "If you come with me, I will try to do that for this particular patient with whom I have had a beautiful relationship for so many years".
>
> On the agreed day, the palliative care physician went with the GP to visit Phil's family. They were very friendly, and the doctors prepared everything. Phil was really at the end of his life. A nurse was already taking care of a syringe driver, and he would have lived for no more than two or three days had euthanasia not been performed. When the GP said goodbye to his patient before giving the injection, Phil said "Doctor, you are my hero!" That was so moving. And after the patient had died, the daughter asked the doctor "Was that all right for you?" That was the first thing she said.

This story shows deep respect and how it can be developed between a doctor and their patient, especially as this is not always the case. Some patients or families can be very forceful. They put a lot of pressure on doctors with statements along the lines of "It is my right" and "I want it and you should do it". However, it does not help. It is not a good way to deal with such requests.

The palliative care physician in the above story does not consider himself a 'euthanastic' (i.e. enthusiastic about euthanasia), but in some situations, as in the hero story, he felt this intervention was in line with what the patient, the family and the doctor wanted. There was a balance. He feels that in some occasions, euthanasia can be seen as good care, provided it is set within a proper relationship with a patient and family, enabling them to discuss treatment options and leaving the final decision to the doctor. Furthermore, every respect is due to a GP or physician who does not want to do it.

There is a form of reciprocity that may come from a relationship between a professional and a patient who is dying and their loved ones. Working at relational depth (Mearns & Cooper, 2005), professional boundaries may become blurred into a shared humanity where being there for each other is healing for the professional as well as the patient. All are human, and all share the burden of loss as well as the reality of our mortality.

Reconciliation with oneself and with others

A Belgian palliative care physician recounted the following story in which, in his judgement, he did not feel there was 'a good death':

> Geoff was in his early fifties and suffered cancer of the lung. He spent many months in the hospice because he had no one to care for him. He had had a

difficult life. His father was in the army and gave Geoff a severe upbringing. As a result, their relationship was poor. A very sensitive child, Geoff was sent to a military school, where he was really broken. Ever since, he has had a life of working a bit, drinking a lot, living on the street for some years, contending with a lot of psychological and even psychiatric problems.

The nurses at the hospice did not feel at ease with him, and so it was difficult. On the other hand, I had a good relationship with him. I found I could relate to a person with love and wisdom, although he had not led a life of wisdom. Sometimes he had really uncontrolled anger, and we could not deal with this in the hospice. I explained to him that I was sorry, but we had to send him to the hospital for a week or two. Then I added that when he had calmed down, he would be welcome to come back to the hospice. He said to me "I will go to the lunatics again", and I replied "No, not the lunatics; It is a place for vulnerable people like you, who have been wounded and made vulnerable by life".

Eventually he came back to the hospice, and discharge home was considered for him in spite of his difficulties. He had a friend, but it was a drinking friend who could not care for him. It was an impossible choice in fact. Eventually Geoff declared, "I will remain at the hospice, and I want euthanasia". He suffered a lot, physical problems but also existential ones: not to have a home, no friends that really cared for him. It was obvious that he suffered, and we could not alleviate it, and it came to a point where we said, "If that is really what you want, you can have euthanasia".

The last day of Geoff's life, his godfather – with whom he had always had a good relationship and who was the responsible person Geoff turned to when he was in trouble – came with his wife, and they stayed with him the whole day. What really shocked me before Geoff died was that he was so negative, saying things like "I have ruined my life", "I was nothing", "I had wrong friends", "I was of no use to anyone".

To this physician, Geoff's passing did not feel like 'a good death'. He felt he had failed Geoff because they had not been able to help him at least to accept himself as the person he was. The doctor had pleaded, saying, "The fact your godfather is still in your life is proof that you mean something to him. You are a person that matters to him". But all the encouragement Geoff received did not help him to see himself as a person that mattered in this life. No one seemed able to help him feel any self-respect. They had many conversations, but they all failed to instil in Geoff a more positive image of himself, and thus euthanasia felt like a negative escape. Even if Geoff had died a natural death or if they had used sedation to alleviate his pain, this would still have felt like a bad death because Geoff was not able, to the last breath, to love or accept himself.

Unconditional acceptance is very important at the end of life. It is a time when people make up their life stories or narratives. They ponder about what was acceptable or what they could have done differently. They evaluate what was right and what was wrong and wonder whether there are things they want to restore, people they want to meet or speak to before they die . . . Some people, like Geoff, can be very severe on themselves, and many need to be reminded to be kind to themselves. If we are personally open to unconditional acceptance, it can create a field of energy that makes it easier for patients to start that process themselves. It is like learning through observation, being an inspiration for the patient. As one of our interviewees said:

> We have to look as caregiver at how we can guide the patient so that they can die peacefully, that they can be satisfied even if life was not perfect. Because life is never perfect and we can always look at the half-empty glass and the half-full glass. So how can we help them to look and see that the glass is not totally empty, and that we can focus also on the things that were superb, excellent and what they did well so that it is not black or white, but something in between?

A palliative care nurse spoke about reconciliation and how she has helped people feel calmer and more peaceful when approaching death. But, she insists, one cannot force it upon them; if they don't want to go there, that is fine too. Reconciliation for her is about meaningful connection; it is about offering the patient and their family some time out in which to focus on what they need with someone from outside who might encourage their communication and understanding of each other. It is about a better emotional and peaceful acceptance of what is about to happen. A palliative care physician remembers Paula very clearly:

> Paula came in with motor neurone disease. She had a very striking look like a benign witch, with a hooked nose and long dark hair combed back. She used to be a poet.
> When Paula came into the hospice she couldn't speak, and she had to be fed by the nurses – a skilled process as getting the food in the right spot so that she could swallow it was tricky. But Paula still had her arms, so she used them to communicate by writing. She was an incredible enthusiast. One would go in and ask her a question, and she would seize a piece of paper and with big looping speedy handwriting she'd be giving lengthy answers. I'd look at it and respond and then she'd be off again. There were sheaves of paper all over the bed.
> And yet Paula kept an inner peace. She had accepted the fact that she was dying. She was a spiritualist, and she talked with a friend of hers at great length about what it would be like when they crossed over. She did not show

any collapse or distress. She held her centre somehow. I don't think she was pretending. She was just so striking, really amazing. I can still see her in my mind's eye, scrawling away, her writing big and bold, like her enthusiastic character. She loved life till the very end.

To this doctor, Paula and her attitude were striking in every sense of the word. He was in awe and remembers her to this day as someone who loved life till the very end and who somehow kept an inner peace and grounding despite the ordeal of the limitations and progression of her illness. To him as an observer, Paula's death thus seemed to be good, because there appeared to be a healing process which led to her being at peace with herself, even if her body was dying.

People's physical illness may be incurable, but their psyche, their relationships and their spirit may be in harmony, reunited. They seem ready to go. Death, after all, is a normal part of life. It's a coming to terms with all those different elements. Maybe it is also about a person having found their purpose in life. They may discover it isn't at all about working long hours in the City but actually spending time with their family or repairing broken relationships. Some people, not necessarily dying, say their cancer was actually a great gift to them. It forced them to reappraise their lives. They might give up their highly stressful, highly paid job and go travelling, volunteer, paint or spend time in nature.

Comfortable, peaceful, free of pain – an ideal death?

As suggested by the chaplain, who challenges this idea in favour of a personal death, many people consider 'a good death' to be a peaceful one, without too many complaints. For the physician, managing to control pain and symptoms with the drugs and techniques at their disposal is a priority. But unfortunately – luckily on very rare occasions – this is not always possible, and patients have to contend with residues of pain and discomfort. This is when some people who believe that death should be clean and comfortable may consider euthanasia as an option. A hospital physician in the Netherlands tells the following sad story of where medical skills fail to give comfort and relieve pain.

Andrew was very strong. He had rectal cancer, which was growing into the sacral bone with lots of nerve involvement and very much pain. I did not know the patient. I was called in by the anaesthetist of the pain management team who was treating Andrew. They could not relieve his pain; even the epidural did not work. We decided to start palliative sedation, but the question was "This guy is so strong, this could go on for weeks". And there could be no discussion about end-of-life care or assisted dying or any other option. We did not know anything about this patient. Even his GP had not been able to talk with him about end of life and treatment options; he simply would not talk about it. Luckily, Andrew died after a few days, but I could see him lying there for weeks with various complications. I always want, if possible, to control the pain with the drugs we have, but sometimes it is not possible.

Every effort was made to bring Andrew to a peaceful and painless end, but sadly, that was beyond even modern medicine. Indeed, this physician feels that, if possible, death should be clean and comfortable, and luckily in these days of advanced medical care, that is often within reach. He has, on rare occasions, practised euthanasia and found that patient and family were happy when he came with the medication. He stays with them until the death. In his experience, Andrew had a really bad death. He fought very hard and died in agony even though he was sedated.

Peace and comfort are not only about physical pain and symptom control. A 'good death' is also when all the caregivers feel well and are not in too much moral distress. Dying is a process one could compare to the playing of a symphony, the quality of which results from the working together of complex physical, emotional, social and spiritual factors of all the people in the orchestra. The same can be said for all the people at the bedside. Not all caregivers, unfortunately, are aware of this, as transpires in the following story:

> In a palliative care reflective practice group a doctor spoke up: "I have a problem. A patient died, and I do not know what he died of". The facilitator asked "And what is the problem? Was it a good death?" "No" the doctor replied, "I did not know what he died of".

This doctor still had to learn that a good death is not one that is good for him, i.e. that he felt confident in knowing what the patient died of, but one that is good for all involved: doctor, patient, family and team. As the group facilitator said, we have to teach physicians to work in a team as well as with patients and their families, who all have their own psychological, emotional, social and spiritual worries. Sometimes working in a team and respecting patients' and families' wishes can be harrowing as the following story reveals.

> There was a conflict on one of the wards where a very young person with Ewing cancer who knew he was dying refused morphine. Anthony only allowed a small dose when he needed to be washed or repositioned; at other times he refused the painkillers, because he said, "I have had a very short life and I feel that when they give me morphine, I become drowsy and I am not myself. I want to remain myself until my death, because I do not have much time".

This was a situation where the nurses protested because for them this was not a good death. For them, a good death had a certain direction, a way the patient goes. As nurses, they expect to administer more and more morphine, and everybody is quiet as they sit round the bed. But Anthony said: "No. It is not what I want, and I do not want to die that way".

Each time they had to work with Anthony, they saw that he was in tremendous pain. Sometimes they pleaded with him to ask for some morphine, but he said "No, I want to stay clearheaded. I need to stay clearheaded". This was very difficult for everybody involved.

Realising the situation was so confronting and painful for the nurses, the chaplain came up with the idea that they could change the rota system. Instead of coming to care for Anthony four days running as was usual, there would be a rota which required them to come to him one day at a time. So while it was difficult, at least they knew that they would not have to come and see him four days running. The ones for whom it was not a problem could maintain the four-day rota if they so wished, but actually, they all chose for the one-day rota because it was so much less painful for them.

In this story, respecting Anthony's request runs contrary to the nurses' training; they all felt they had to DO something. To give medication is what they learned to do when they see somebody in pain. One of the less developed aspects in health care – and more generally in modern Western society – is the area where there is nothing to be done, where the only possible thing is simply to be fully present and to listen. Usually it is about listening to questions which one cannot solve or answer or which, by definition, have no answers. This is something that many health care workers find difficult to deal with, because they want to DO something. When a patient says they are in pain, it does not necessarily mean that they experience physical pain. It may be heartache or loss, fear or whatever. So "I have pain" does not mean "Where are the painkillers?" This issue is quite often forgotten or misunderstood in the immediate moment.

Being prepared

About 80% of people die a natural death, and the doctor, nurse or family may not always be there. Many people in nursing homes, for instance, die quietly and easily, sometimes in their sleep, or they get pneumonia and die in a slow way. Often when a loved one is in a nursing home, the family realises that they are old, vulnerable and frail, which makes the advent of death more natural for them.

At other times, death can involve great pain and a sense of loneliness, helplessness and fear of what the next few hours or weeks may hold. And when it comes to a decision along the lines of 'OK, let's allow death now', it usually takes some time for patient and loved ones to adjust to the inevitable, and the physician, nurses and other caregivers need to talk a lot about the processes and consequences, sometimes over a number of days. Preparing the team and family for that kind of event has everything to do with communication and compassion!

We saw in Andrew's story how difficult it was for the hospital physician and the GP to have a conversation with Andrew about what his medical future might hold. Andrew would not go there, and this had to be respected. This lack of real communication may have contributed to the doctor's feeling that Andrew's was not a good death. Several, if not all, of our interviewees stressed how important it is to build a relationship with the patient and their family. This comes with time and through deepening conversations about their condition, treatment options and what can be expected, thus contributing to patient's and family's preparedness. Sadly, sometimes, time pressures force the outcome in this important aspect. A palliative care physician shared:

> I was asked to go and see somebody who had just been admitted as an emergency and was very close to death. He was obviously acutely distressed, very short of breath, with a huge amount of pain, gasping and in extremis. His family was sitting around him in complete shock and horror. I could feel the atmosphere of the horror in there, very dark, bleak, bitter and overwhelming. I gave the patient injections of painkillers and tranquillisers to relieve his distress. That worked. I could see him calming down and settling. He died not long afterwards. The family, however, was left in a kind of horrified traumatic trance.

This doctor had managed to relieve the patient's distress, but he did not have enough time to prepare the family and to get the patient comfortable early enough so that patient and family could spend time together quietly and say their goodbyes. To him and to them, it was a difficult death experience.

There are different aspects to preparedness. It can be about time to build a relationship and/or to relieve a patient's pain and distress in order to give the patient and family, as well as staff, the opportunity to talk about what is to come, spend time together quietly and say their goodbyes. It can also be about openness, capacity and readiness to talk about these matters. Some will express feelings and fears; others may find it difficult to engage with themselves and each other on a territory where people can feel very vulnerable. Furthermore, cultural differences can have a huge impact on people's feelings and expressions at this critical time.

A 'good death' is when patients have their needs and wishes respected. The first level of this is, of course, pain and symptom control, but underneath that, a 'good death' has to do with sharing the process. It sometimes occurs that, if staff and relatives have not explored the idea of death in their own life, they cannot share it with others. Some people are not even able to think about death, and hence, a lot of prejudice around dying is brought about by ignorance.

A palliative care support team in a university hospital has made it a priority to talk with relatives so as to at least inform them, if not involve them, in what is going on. Their experience is that whatever the treatment options, the adjustment of patient and family are greatly improved by open and pro-active communication about what they might expect. This puts a strain on the team, but they feel it is well worth it for all involved. A psychologist noted how they try to encourage conversation at this important time:

> Some people may say, "In my family we never talk about these things" and we will reply by asking, "Do you think it is important?" . . . "I think it is". . . . "Do you want to give it a try?"

Similarly, with the professionals in the hospital.

> For the last three years the team has had increasing involvement with the intensive care unit. They now consider such questions as 'What kind of family is this?', 'What is their culture?' and try to help and prepare families accordingly. For example, there are huge differences in how a Jewish family, an East European one or a West European one think about death and dying.

With the help of the palliative care support team, people working in the intensive care unit now consider their role more as accompanying the dying process and looking at how they can make the turning point together, thus making it easier for the patient and family.

Some assumptions which colour our perception

Dying is a very individual process. All sorts of efforts may have been made to avoid the experience or postpone it, but whatever is done, someday, it occurs. Death is both universal for all living creatures and plants and also unavoidable. People respond to this reality in endlessly varied ways which are guided by the assumptions they make to a certain extent.

In the last section, we discussed the notion of 'a good death' in all its variability. Now we will consider the way humans use their personal resources and beliefs such as their sense of autonomy, status and previous experience in coping with this potential radical change and how a person's feelings are raided by major illness and impending death.

Some people are very fearful or forceful regarding the Great Unknown, others are phlegmatic, and some even approach the situation in a relaxed mood and with humour. We are all born in different circumstances, we lead varied lives, and we die so. In this section we review people's responses to the challenges of serious illness. We also note the response of the families and friends and, indeed, the medical profession itself. Rarely do people enjoy being seriously ill, but when they are so affected, they frequently (sometimes with help) find resources of character which they had not previously recognised. Thus, through the trial of a crisis, a new aid for the future is mobilised. Such discoveries can reduce the fears and doubts of patients and family, thus enabling a new positive outlook.

Medicine as an art and science has much to offer, while many people sense it as a threat, but it can also be the key to a new outlook which impacts a person's approach to their life and their death.

Self-determination and longevity set against euthanasia

Most people think autonomy is very important, and that can be a reason a patient may ask for euthanasia. They do not want to be a burden on the family. Mathilde, a mother of four middle-aged children, who is alive and kicking, made the following comment:

> I have read in the newspaper that life in a nursing home costs £4000 a month, and my pension is £2000 a month. So, when I look at my savings, this means that I can afford a nursing home for 5 years. Her son replied, "What kind of calculation are you making? Who says that you will have to go into a nursing home in the first place? Secondly, we are here, and as a family, we can provide for you". She said "No, no, no, I don't want to be dependent on anybody. I don't want to be a bother to anybody".

This is a very strange priority in our contemporary society. Yet it is so true for so many people. For a hospital physician in the Netherlands, it is important that people do not ask for euthanasia because they want to die but because they have so many complaints that it is impossible to live any longer as a free and responsible person. In the latter situation, he thinks it can be a good solution. The following patient illustrates this.

> Paul was suffering very badly. Lots of complaints. Nothing worked. He was in a really bad condition. He had a very close family and didn't want to leave it, but at the same time, he said, "I can't go on any longer and would like to have euthanasia". So, we started the process, and he was very happy that we could stop the suffering.

Paul would have died in a few weeks. They could have given him palliative sedation, which is aimed at symptom control not at causing death. But this physician does not want the patient to die from palliative sedation. When deciding to administer it, he expects that the patient will die anyway from the progression of the disease, in a few days, hopefully.

Another physician reports that many people who ask for euthanasia prepare for it as if it was a form of insurance. Those who proceed with it are people who want to keep their autonomy till the last day and do not want the unpredictability of the end of life. For instance, when people cannot go to the toilet by themselves, they might say, "That is not what I want". There is an issue in keeping control and organising the dying process. Euthanasia is a way to 'do' something and avoid helplessness.

While some people seem to revere autonomy per se, others may find meaning in living with someone's lack of autonomy, as the following story illustrates.

> Patrick had a terrible car accident and was left completely vegetative. He couldn't move nor say anything, but he was alive. Patrick came back to his parents' home and stayed there for 15 years. His mother was absolutely dedicated to continuing Patrick's life, and she nursed him wonderfully and carefully.
>
> When people said, "There is no life there; he is as good as dead", she got terribly angry. "How can you say that?" She fought for his survival until eventually he died naturally. For our interviewee and many others, this was a horrific thing to witness. Patrick's mother would take visitors to his room, saying, "Talk to him". It virtually destroyed her. She died shortly after her son's death.

What moved this lady to care for her son in this way? What was the discomfort of the visitors? What sense could they make of Patrick's situation and life? Like so many others who are living in prolonged coma, Patrick asks us questions for which we have no answers. Our feelings, beliefs and opinions will differ and clash, as one cannot remain indifferent in the face of such appalling suffering and mystery. As one of our interviewees light-heartedly put it:

> I am not sure that just going for longevity of life is worthwhile in society. I quite like the way the Indians do it: Granddad is pretty useful as long as he can chop the kindling and if he is no good, he is put out on the pavement and he dies quite quickly because he has no purpose.

This reminds us that purpose in life is important, however one understands that. Patrick's mum found purpose in caring for him; the Indian granddad loses his evident use when he no longer contributes to the family.

Living with unpredictability

Two of the most fundamental realities in life, our beginning and our ending, are events over which we as individuals have little or no control. Our parents bring us to life; we do not have a choice. Similarly, we cannot choose not to die. However, people want to be able to take control over how and when death happens; some even consider it a right. A hospice chaplain shared his dealing with these questions, trying to verbalise people's assumptions:

> Lots of people assume that we have to die in pain. I have never seen anybody die in the hospice screaming out in pain, because the development in medication has been so phenomenal that it has become very rare that anyone needs to suffer that degree of pain. If they are in considerable pain, we give them something more. We recognise that the side effect may be that it will knock them out a bit, but they look peaceful, they look calm, they look relaxed and they slip away. A lot of this is about verbalising fears and anxieties, and one can turn that into having a conversation about what is going on and the questions people have about the nature of death and dying and about their destiny.
>
> Sometimes we can get into that journey in a very serious, deep way, and sometimes we can meet a person who has had enough about talking about these things as well. In the right relationship when someone says "I want to die", I might say something like "Well, we have a very dim view about queue jumpers in this place. You have to jolly well wait in the queue". And they have a laugh. And suddenly they are reduced from this big existential statement to something more human that you can engage in that moment.
>
> At other times, when talking with people, it is just humour. I will never use it flippantly, but it releases tension. I had a conversation with this lady who is very much a person of faith. I said, "You know what? We all want to go to heaven, but we just don't want to die to get there. . . " So she laughed at that and said, "Yes, it is true, and we are fearful of not knowing the way there".
>
> To another patient, I said: "You know what the difference is between you and me? We are on the same road, but probably you are on the outside lane. Maybe I'm in the inside lane, maybe I'm in the far lane. I don't know. But the point is we are all on the same road. We are dying, we just don't know when. I hope that I can find somebody to walk with me when, like you, I feel frightened and unsure and confused. I am sitting in this position now with you, but I don't know whether I will be in your position next week or in the next month. I just don't know. So rather than worry about that, all that I can do is just to try to live today. And so be present for you here and now".

This chaplain finds ways of breaking the loneliness that stems from the powerlessness to control what is unpredictable. He can meet the patients where they are and share humanity and laughter with them. Something of the fear of death is removed. It ceases to be an ogre. The reality is relieved, but it is still accepted for what its place is in the ultimate experience, for every creature, including us, must die.

Sense of time

It will surprise no one that since there are so many different beliefs about death and dying, including ignorance, it can be difficult to understand each other, let alone reach an agreement about difficult decisions around the bedside of a dying person. When counselling families of the very ill and the bereaved, we have witnessed heightened emotions and confusion in those difficult circumstances. Members of a family, however close they may be, react to death, dying and bereavement in their own very personal ways, and they may find it difficult to respect each other in their grief reactions. A person who is very sad can be shocked by another family member's apparent absence of grief or their denial of what is happening.

People need to both confront and avoid their grief. Research (Stroebe & Shut, 1999) has shown that more resilient individuals can move back and forth between these different states of mind without experiencing great tension, guilt or anxiety. It can be helpful to warn family members that this is likely to happen and encourage them to respect one another's grief process, which will develop along their own personal timeline. A psychologist reported:

> My dad passed away last year, and we took care of him in our house during the last three months of his life. I expected that at some point he would ask for euthanasia, but when the moment came, I was not prepared at all. The euthanasia turned out to be a very clear deadline that enabled me to take some steps towards my father.
>
> We had had a very rough ride. There were even years that we did not have any contact because of everything that happened. In the last months, we tried to reach out to each other, but it did not work. When there was a date and an hour for the euthanasia, all of a sudden there was the deep realisation 'this is the last day of my father's life'. If you want to say things to him, now is the time. It is now or never.
>
> This might sound bizarre, but thanks to the prospect of euthanasia, all of a sudden, my heart opened up, and we had this real deep connection. I said some things to him. He didn't say anything. He just looked at me and touched me. This was a really deep connection that we never had had in our entire life as father and son.
>
> Without the euthanasia, my father would have slipped into a coma, and we wouldn't have had this contact. For my father, there was no escape anymore. He was busying himself day in day out with crosswords, even when he did no longer have the strength to write the words down. It was very threatening for him to get in touch with his emotions. Euthanasia was

another form of escaping. My talking to him was one moment where we got into another dimension or another level, but he could not keep going at that level.

We were both blocked towards each other, which caused deep pain, and we needed extreme measures to open up through that pain. But that I could talk, and that he was open to listen to me, meant a lot. I felt very grateful that we had this moment together, but why did it take so long to get there? And now that we had this moment together, he is no longer there. It had a huge impact on my grieving. Had we not experienced that moment, it would have been even more difficult to say goodbye.

Everything has different sides to it. There is a chance in everything, even in euthanasia, the deadline of which enabled connection between this father and son.

Looking forward to an unknown future

One of our consultants told the following powerful story, illustrating how one's understanding of a situation can influence its outcome, even in circumstances of life and death.

Tom was one of four children. Only towards the end of our school career together did I discover that my friend Tom had porphyria (a life-limiting illness) and was not expected to live until 16. When I was 12, I remember having a really good discussion with my mother about my concern for Tom: "Why is he going to die? He is far too young".

Tom's mum and dad were fantastic, and Tom went on to a leading English boarding school. Although everybody knew Tom was going to die, he had a completely normal education, and his parents paid for it. They were investing in his future, and I think, because they did that, he lived so much longer than was expected.

Tom's parents invested in his future, an investment which speaks of their valuation of his life. This transpired in their attitude personally and financially towards him as a person, however short or long Tom's life expectancy would be. It is our interviewee's belief that this very attitude of his parents contributed to prolonging Tom's life beyond what was expected.

One person who has spent a lot of time with Buddhists, travelling the Himalaya mountains, told us about a very striking difference in perception between Eastern and Western attitudes to death.

When somebody dies in a rocky country such as the Himalayas, you cannot dig a hole in the ground to put them into because you cannot dig the hole. So when people die, their bodies are burned. People in the Himalayas believe they send the spirits up to God, and God will look after them. They, therefore, have a very cheerful optimistic outlook: when they die, they are going up to God, and they will be cared for. So if you talk to a Buddhist in Nepal about dying, they are not at all frightened of dying; they're going up. In the Western world, we dig a hole and put the dead body in it – a much less attractive destiny.

I think simple things like that colour our judgement about how awful death is. You go to a funeral, and people are all dressed in black for an occasional solemnity. My mother was buried, which was simply dreadful. When my father died, I absolutely insisted that he should be cremated. The positivity of that was liberating, a significant contrast to my mother, who is still down there under the ground physically. The Buddhists have a very good approach to death, and I am pretty certain that if you were to go to Nepal, you would find that their view of helping people in extremis is very positive.

If you could mix Buddhism and Christianity, you would have a very good recipe. Buddhists take everything on the chin. They say, "This is what is coming my way, and I will deal with it. If it is one of a million God wishes that I am going to die, I am going to die, but I am going to a better place". Whereas we as a society are terrified of admitting the finality and even the process of death itself.

People's attitude to death depends on the nature of their life experiences. People who live in great poverty may expect death to be better than life. They die with the hope of gain not loss. One's outlook on life will colour their expectations, as this gentleman sums up with some humour:

> Dying is like reading a novel, but you will never finish the last page. You die on the penultimate page, and it is so annoying, because you just want to know who married who, what happened, but you will never know. It is nothing to be frightened about, but you might be cross about that.

The question we cannot answer

Sometimes doctors make death a more fearful process than it need be. They raise expectations by saying, "Take these pills and you'll be cured". The patient hopes for a magic cure, and when they get worse their anxieties soar. "Why am I not responding to these pills?" But actually, in some instances, it is much fairer to say to the patient "There is nothing that I can do here which will really cure you, but we can do things to make life easier".

As a palliative care physician mentioned, the dominant healing paradigm in medicine at present takes a mechanistic approach, seeing the human body as an engine that needs to be put right when it goes wrong. However, it is much more complex than that. Seeing healing as wholeness is richer, since it includes not only the physical body but also psychological, relational, spiritual and ecological aspects. This was exactly Dame Cicely Saunders's point when she talked about 'total pain', by which she meant physical, mental, social and spiritual pain (Saunders, 1964).

We looked at an authoritative textbook of palliative medicine recently (Bruera et al., 2015). About 70% to 80 % was about symptom control, that is, physically based. About 15% to 20 % was on psychological issues. But in a book more than 1,000 pages long, spiritual issues got only three or four pages. The idea that spiritual pain may be connected with and aggravate physical pain seems to have faded in palliative medicine. So despite what Dame Cicely was saying, palliative medicine is getting more medicalised, perhaps because it is easier to concentrate on, or see everything as, symptoms to be controlled by medication.

The things of the spirit are those factors in our experience which seem to have no obvious physical reality, for instance falling in love, developing a proper ambition or noticing the poor and the disheartened around us. We want here to consider some of the questions at the twilight of life that can be regarded as spiritual pain, as expressed in "Why do I have to suffer?", "My heart is broken", "I really failed that person" and other forms of guilt and shame.

Why do we have to suffer?

With the whole process of secularisation in our Western world some phenomena around the deathbed have become taboo because they do not fit easily within the materialistic scientific paradigm of today. People, even people who have been atheist all their life, are wondering what death is about, yet we often miss the openness to address these issues. A Belgian psychologist in palliative care we interviewed – call him Sven – says:

> In my country, we have this wave of professionalism. We want to be taken seriously by medicine. We want to be a branch of medicine. That is not bad, but it has a flip side to it. What I see is that the existential and spiritual dimensions are approached more and more as if we were talking about pain and symptom control. If someone is anxious, we have this pill, if someone is depressed, there is this medication; existential pain . . . we also have palliative sedation. "Why do people have to suffer?" is a question that is heard frequently, as if suffering is a synonym for inhumanity.

Research states that in about 90% of the cases cancer pain can be reduced to acceptable levels (Carlson, 2016). Many health care professionals have a clear view of what physical pain is. But when people start talking about situational pain and spiritual pain which affect their feelings, they wonder what that is. If you cannot touch or see it, it does not exist. Interested in what themes come up at the end of life, Sven sees it as his mission to develop the existential (or essentially human) and the spiritual dimension of palliative care. He reports:

> In this part of the world, there is the Catholic stream and the Humanistic stream. These people do, of course, great work, but there is something missing. Not everyone who has abandoned Christianity finds what they need in Humanism. We need to discover a platform where we can find each other despite the differences, and that is what I am searching for.
>
> We have worked on a project interviewing 6 patients in the last stages of their lives. We asked them, "What things are on your mind at this moment? What deep questions are bothering you now?" In doing so, we revealed the existential and spiritual dimension in order to make those ideas more realistic and practical to the health care professionals.

Sven is sensitive to the fact that in 'secularising' health care chaplaincy, the existential and spiritual questions that people struggle with at the end of life need to find a new language, a different way of being addressed. These spiritual factors are having trouble gaining credibility because they cannot be tested and validated. They are intuitive. Yet when given a chance, people can and are keen to talk about them, as Sven commented:

> It is interesting how with some patients the interviewer in the project managed to talk about things that had never come up in conversations the patient had with the health care professional. This was an eye opener for the professional carer, and I have been able to use it in training, as it has all to do with authenticity and the dangers of the professional mask. There is much interest for this training programme from the first-line carers and volunteers. Unfortunately, the further you go up the ladder, the more obscure and hidden becomes the priority of these matters.

Sven's experience confirms that of a psychiatrist teaching at the Royal Academy of Medicine (Proot & Yorke, 2014, pp. 83–84). He sent medical students off to the wards where they had been working for a couple of weeks to ask a patient two sorts of questions. The first was: "What keeps you going when things are difficult? What are your sources of strength, courage, hope, etc.? How do you deal with adversity? Where do you go for help with that?" The second question was, "Do you think of yourself in anyway as religious or spiritual?" Almost all of the patients said: "Nobody has ever asked me about this before".

The medical students were amazed at the depth and extent of connection they experienced with some of the patients around whose beds they had stood more than once without a hint of anything beyond their pathology,

symptoms and complaints. Similarly, the patients felt honoured and enliv-
ened at being given that space to be who they were. They no longer felt like
children who were bossed about according to medical orders; who they
really were as a person had become significant for this 'doctor' who came to
ask them about their life's experience.

The first set of questions offered a way into exploring patients' inner
resources and strengths and the practical and emotional external support
available to them. The second question opened a door to their spiritual
dimension and sense of being a person and not just a sick body, thus meeting the confusion patients tend to experience when feeling ill without understanding why.

Limitations of the scientific method

Ben, a head of psycho-social and spiritual care in a hospice, recognises that
existential and spiritual issues are not easily talked about, even in training, and that addressing these questions suffers from presuppositions and
prejudices. When training, he starts off with looking at the strengths and
limitations of the tools people use, whether he is talking to nurses, medics,
psychologists or physiotherapists. He suggests:

> I ask a very simple question: "What are the two basic questions behind the
> scientific method?" Much if not most of the scientific method comes out
> in the questions "What?" and "How?": What is going on here? How do we
> understand that? What is happening for the patient? How do we treat them?
> What is happening when this patient's blood count goes down? How do we
> respond to that?
>
> What? How? . . . The philosophical root of the scientific method is radi-
> cal materialism. It has its proper place and can be very useful. We look
> through a set of lenses, and whatever we can actually see and measure,
> that can be taken as a given. This is evidence, and this is evidence-based
> practice.
>
> But what about the other issues? When a patient comes into the office
> of the oncologist for test results and hears, "I'm really sorry, but you have
> aggressive lung cancer with secondaries in your brain and bones", what is the
> first question that patient asks? . . . "Why?" Exactly. In the hospice, we try to
> hold the 'how?' and 'what?', together with the 'why?' As soon as we throw
> out the 'why?', we have lost something very important.
>
> The 'why?' question is when people ask: "Why me?", "Why does this
> happen to me?" But there are other things as well which cannot be meas-
> ured by the scientific method. Things like love, meaning, music, art . . . In
> music for instance, all you see is a bunch of notes on a piece of paper. So,
> if someone is going to count the number of notes, this particular work

has 5.386 notes, eight notes which are repeated in various ways for 5.386 times, or whatever it is. Have we actually grasped what the music is in that way? No, we have not. We have lost something very basic, very precious. The same happens with meaning. How do we construct meaning? What is a sense of justice? Is your sense of justice the same as that of terrorist fighters?

There are so many things which expand beyond the limitations of the scientific method. One can be a good doctor by knowing how to work with the scientific method, but they will be a better doctor if they understand the limitations of the scientific method and that human beings do not only live according to radical materialism. When, for example, people marry or choose a partner, they are not going to measure their partner by the scientific method, because it is something highly personal. It is the internal world which measures and gives value, meaning to that person.

Unfortunately, one of us has come across a doctor who, when asked a 'why?' question, replied, "I do not deal with 'why?', I only deal with 'what?' and 'how?'". When he was told about this, Ben sighed . . . In Christianity, he said, we talk about the ten commandments – 'Thou shalt, thou shalt not' – and what we keep on hearing from the scientific method is 'Thou shalt not ask why!'

Research (Fitch & Bartlett, 2019; Hatamipour et al., 2015; Puchalski et al., 2009) found that most patients in palliative care expect the medical team to pay attention to their spiritual needs, yet doctors and nurses usually wait for the patient to take the initiative to address this topic. The challenge for the future is to encourage patients to talk about their significant relationships with their caregivers and to train physicians and nurses in addressing the spiritual dimension of care. To have a total picture of the patient and their relationships, their values, their existential framework and life story is important, both when deciding on a person-centred treatment plan and when discussing end-of-life care, including treatment options and requests for euthanasia and palliative sedation.

The story behind the patient

One of the ways by which we can have an inkling of a response to the 'why?' question is by having an ear for the story behind the patient. A palliative care researcher, Myriam, told this moving story:

It was suggested that we should visit Mark, an 88-year-old man, for our research. His GP gave us his contact details while saying, "This is Mark's address, but if you don't find him there he will be at the building across the road where his girlfriend lives". I went to Mark's address and rang the bell. There was nobody, so I remembered the warning and went over the road. He was there, together with a lady in her eighties. Mark had a terminal renal cell carcinoma.

When patients consented for this study, one of the criteria was that they had to realise they were in end-of-life care. When I came to talk to Mark, he denied it. I asked him, "What do you know about your disease?" and he said, "I have something in my kidney, but I am going to be ok". That really surprised me.

Later I went to see Mark for the second time. This was around noon, and he was in his own home. I saw that he had laid a few photos on the table. We did the survey, and then Mark said, "Do you have some time? Would you like a cup of coffee?" I said I would love one. "I have some photos for you" he said, and he showed them to me. They were photos from the world war when he was a soldier, and he said, "I will tell you a story.

"When I was 17 or 18, I was in love with a girl, her name was Rose and we wanted to marry. But our parents had to agree and when they came together, we were waiting in the kitchen while the parents were in the living room. They had a long conversation. After a while we went to see them. They said we could not marry because Rose's parents were not wealthy enough to pay for the wedding". Mark said, "My heart broke and we each went our own way". Then came the war, and Mark found another wife, who he married, had five children, and they were happy together.

When Mark was 70 years old, his wife had passed away, and he had to go to the hospital for a fracture to his leg. He said, "I was walking in the hospital corridor with my physiotherapist, and looking to the left, I saw Rose and we recognised each other". By that time, she too was a widow, and after 60 years, Rose and Mark met each other again in that hospital. It was amazing, but it really happened.

Rose was the lady across the road, because when they met each other again, they decided to live together. This was now 16 years ago. Mark denied his palliative stage because he said, "We take it day by day. We have waited for each other for 60 years, and now we have been together for 15 years, and we want to cherish every day. We do not want to think about the rest. We will see". So that is why he did not want to talk about whether he was in end of life or not.

Having heard this amazing story, Myriam understood better why Mark would not own up to his palliative condition. Knowing the story behind the patient, we may be in a better position to appreciate how they think or why they decide something. Without that, we can wonder why they take a third-line chemotherapy, but we don't understand their reasons. If we know their story and can comprehend their reasons, we can better understand them and guide them in their care.

Myriam was surprised by the warm welcome she received from patients she met for the research. Meetings were not limited to applying the tool and doing the survey. Coffee was served afterwards, and the spouse or children also came in, so the visit became a social event. These were very intimate moments with patients, who were very open with the researchers. The stories told were amazing. And when they visited for the second time, they were expected, so the stories were even more detailed and emotional. Although it was confronting at times, Myriam's experience of these conversations was very positive. It changed her view on end-of-life care, and it even changed her view on her personal life to a degree. The trajectory of her research became life changing.

Fears, stresses and strains

In an earlier passage, we recognised the importance of personal resources and having the capacity to use them in difficult or threatening circumstances like being told that one had a major illness or that one was close to death. Our resources are not the only gift that helps us to cope or, in misuse, to flounder. Our feelings are fundamental to the way we relate to ourselves and to other people and clearly with the difficulties of life.

Yet here again, the picture is not straightforward, for there are parts of us which we are happy to make public where we feel able to share what we feel. On the other side, we have feelings we can hardly recognise or accept for ourselves. They are hidden under lock and key, but in certain circumstances, they can emerge and influence a situation. Moreover, the boundary between the two parts can also be blurred and behaviour, outlook and self-esteem undermined. We cease to be whole or 'together' people.

Situations of stress, threat, rivalry and loss can act as keys to releasing feelings which create confusion. They are muddled for us and, when expressed, misunderstood by others. Relationships understandably become taut. In difficult times, it is easy to feel helpless and alone, but it is not necessary if we can recognise and manage the boundary between our two sides.

Being a burden

Many people fear being a burden. One becomes a burden from the day one is sick, but dependency also creates a way of allowing people to help and to give something back. Caring for someone is not a problem as long as we do not force people to care for us in a way that is not acceptable to them. A GP on the Continent told us that many patients would request euthanasia out of fear of becoming a burden to their loved ones. Some people, he says, just do not want to live these last days of their life. They do not find any meaning in them, whilst their close families are liable to become stressed and exhausted as they care for them. The following story of a patient–doctor dialogue is telling:

> Gerard told me that on the day of his diagnosis he really thought about suicide. He told me in front of his wife that he considered suicide and that the only reason he did not do it was because his family would have all the problems of dealing with the police and so on. . .
>
> Diagnosis took away some of the meaning of his life. His resources were independence, including being able to go to his holiday home with a much-loved orchard. He felt that because of his disease he would get dependent on other people, and that made it too hard for him to carry on.

A parallel to the patient feeling a burden can be found in the family and/or the doctor wondering whether they have done all they could. An oncologist told us the following story:

> Lionel was in hospital because his bowels did not work anymore due to his colon cancer. Chemotherapy did not improve his condition. One morning I had a discussion with Lionel, saying that it was pointless to continue with chemotherapy because of his worsening condition. I told him that there was no more we could do, and I expected him to live for a few weeks.
>
> Then I asked him where he would like to go, what he would like to do. Given the choice, would he rather stay in the hospital or be going home? His wife said, "I'm very busy with the shop. Furthermore, some people can help, but only for a short time". There was also the possibility of going to a hospice.
>
> In the same discussion, I brought up the subject of him not going into intensive care or DNAR (Do Not Attempt Resuscitation). I told him that because we had no possible way to treat the cancer, it did not make sense to tackle irreversible consequences of the disease. I asked Lionel how he thought we should treat his symptoms when they got worse. Would we have to start palliative sedation? What were his thoughts about euthanasia?"
>
> Lionel had never thought about hospice or dying before, so I asked him to think about those options, and we could talk further the next day. He knew his condition was getting worse. He had a lot of complaints, nausea . . . The consequence was that we could not change it and that his time to live was about two weeks. This came as a shock, and a hard one, for the patient and his family.

What is striking in this story is its humanity. We can put ourselves in Lionel's position. He struggles to find answers to the questions posed to him by the doctor. His wife clearly found it difficult to cope with the idea of him being at home for perfectly good reasons. An autopsy after Lionel's death revealed lots of tumours in the lungs. The family were relieved to hear that it was so bad, because in their grieving, they were wondering whether they had done enough and whether there might have been another, more positive way forward.

Death, a defeat?

Earlier, we told the story of Geoff, who was not able, to the last breath, to love or accept himself even though his godfather had come to see him on the day he was euthanised. Geoff's physician was surprised that, after 20 years in palliative care, he could still be confronted with a situation which troubled him for quite a long time. As he said, "No system of medicine or care has all the answers, because we do not have the answers to the ultimate question of death itself".

More generally, many medical doctors long to save lives, and to them, all kinds of dying can be understood as a defeat. Their attitude differs a lot. Some are not interested even to cooperate with the palliative care team. They say "This is your job". They refer the patient on to another specialty, i.e. palliative care, when they can no longer save a patient's life. Others want to be alongside the patient all along their journey. They want to do it well and ask for the help of the palliative care team.

A psychologist in a palliative care support team on the Continent shared how people's hopes and expectations are raised by the research mission of their university hospital:

> When treatment is pursued in a university hospital, it is because the doctors want to do good for the patient and the family. The immediate focus of the palliative care team, therefore, can be on what is important, and we have conversations with the medical team along the lines of "Have you discussed this decision with the family?" "No. Is it important to discuss this?" "Yes".
>
> On the other hand, for families and patients, going to the university hospital means it is serious, the situation is critical, it is 'bad news'. But also, patients and families come setting all their hopes and expectations on the university's capacity to help them. The corollary of that is that patients' expectations are higher. This has huge implications for the palliative care team when patients and families get very angry when they are being told nothing more can be done.

Unfortunately, a lot of time is being wasted. Doctors may push for more and more treatment and postpone talking to the patient about their vulnerability and the limitations of the therapeutic trajectory. They talk along the lines of "This treatment could give you one more year" but do not ask "What quality of life do you hope for?" Similarly, patients who are in a research project may feel they have no right or reason to communicate about their thoughts and feelings and express them. They feel they have to be grateful to be given this opportunity and be a good patient. They think they have nothing to say, but actually, they have a lot to contribute. Far from them being just a dummy for the research, they are speaking, thinking and feeling subjects and, as such, could help the research and the researcher.

Whether wanting more and more treatments – on the part of the patient and/or on the part of the doctors – is likely to have to do with unrealistic hope for a cure or fear of failure, the magic does not always work, and some doctors may find it difficult to accept that. They may wait too long to broach the subject of end of life, often until there is no other alternative, and then suddenly being told there is no more that can be done can be shattering for the patient.

The palliative care support team is called in at a critical moment in the career of a patient. They come to ask the patient whether they want to go home or to a hospice. They are involved with the family, considering the end-of-life options and walking alongside them until the end.

Learning from experience

It is not uncommon in health care that people can be very supportive of and respectful towards a patient but also be very severe on themselves and with their colleagues. The proximity of death puts stress on the boundaries we create throughout our lives and raises issues of which we are not even conscious. If we can consider 'healing' or reconciliation as becoming whole again, it is equally important not to wait with the healing process until we are nearly dead. Sven tries to open a space for this with nurses and caregivers. He recounts the experiential learning he gives:

> Some really had to hurry to come to the training course and found it difficult to focus. I invited them to make themselves comfortable and take the time to ask the question, "How am I doing right now? How am I? Right here, right now. Let's give careful attention to that". Some became really emotional, others very angry: "What are you doing here? You are touching deep layers, and we don't want that".
>
> They could experience firsthand the emotions they have anyway. They carry them around. I could tell them that people who go into burnout are not the people who are in touch with their emotions; they are those who try to build a wall between the patients and themselves. So I taught them how to handle these emotions whenever they emerge.

It can be surprising that people who work with end-of-life patients day in and day out react in such a way. Many people are not used to making space for and talking about their emotions. Even more, in some professions (firemen, surgeons, paramedics, soldiers. . .) people need to pretend they have no emotions in order to deal with what they have to do for their jobs or professions. They are trained to defend themselves psychologically, and they need to do it because they lack time to process the emotions as they emerge. The Grenfell fire disaster is a good example. It is not uncommon in group dynamics addressing emotions that people react in similar ways, saying, for instance, "My company is paying big money for this course and what you are suggesting is not good enough. I can do that on the train". Sven continues:

> In our existential and spiritual care training, we build up the intensity of the exercises, and we then come to doing the dying exercise. We put mattresses on the ground, and people lie down, with a blanket over them. We instruct them to imagine that they are in the last hour of their life − it is important to create the right atmosphere with dimmed lights, the right focus and the right attention − and then we say, "You are about to die, but you can have a conversation with one person before you die. Who will it be? What are you going to say?"
>
> People get really emotional. It is, of course, an 'as if' exercise, but it seems very real, and they get in touch with what it could be like to die for them. It is a magnificent lesson for them in the present, and we experience that people make some choices in their lives after that sort of exercise: "I have never seen it that clear, and this is what I am going to do".
>
> We try to work with a mix of people from different religions, different philosophy, creating a rich environment in which we can learn from each other. If I am really convinced that there is an afterlife, what can I learn from someone who does not have that belief and vice versa? We never try to convince people. What we try to do is to create respect and openness for one another so that we can also have this openness towards the patient.

This experience shows how creating safety and security in caregivers around death and dying enhances their openness towards the patient. They never forget the experience on the floor, and many frequently recall it when they are in the actual circumstance with another person dying.

Asked whether, in training, he could involve doctors and help them recognise what they feel in response to what they see in the bed and put their scientific approach into context, Sven replied:

> I do train doctors, though not enough. I wish I could see them more. In supervision, nine times out of ten, it is the doctor who is not present. Sometimes in our training, we have a few doctors, but those who come are nearly always the junior ones, or they already have this open mind.

For me spirituality and science are not two different worlds. You can approach spirituality in a scientific way. Of course, it is limited, but you can do it. For instance, when I talk to an audience of doctors about the near-death experience and what the importance of that might be for palliative care, I usually get these very critical questions by which they try to push me over. That is when I am grateful for my scientific background, and they are startled. "This guy knows about methodology and randomised control . . . yet he is talking about deathbed experience, what is happening here?"

What I am trying to do is to build bridges. I have a foot in both worlds, I know more or less what it is about. If I say I did a vision quest and this and that happened to me, this is a scientific statement in the sense that you can falsify it, but to falsify it, you have to do a vision quest. I am not putting my energy into people who say "that is not the case" if they are not willing to go into the experience. It is like someone who says "music does not move people", but they do not want to listen to music. That is an endless discussion. You only have a right to speak if you are doing it yourself.

Understanding and experience involves clear participation, and these examples show what a huge impact this can have on the quality of end-of-life care and on the well-being of all involved.

To go further. . .

1   What are my beliefs and expectations about death and dying? Where do they stem from?
2   In palliative care, 'the ill person and their family' is the patient. What would I be sensitive to or look out for: physically? Psychologically? Socially? Spiritually? How would I attend to those needs?
3   How will I make the most of working multi-professionally at the end of life?

Acknowledgements

Text extracts from Proot, C. & Yorke, M., *Life to Be Lived: Challenges and Choices for Patients and Carers in Life-threatening Illnesses*, Oxford University Press, Oxford, UK, Copyright © 2014, reproduced with permission of the Licensor through PLSclear.

Notes

1 For more information, we refer to the WHOQOL: Measuring Quality of Life (World Health Organization, 2018), the Supportive and Palliative Care Indicators

tool (The University of Edinburg, 2010) and the Palliative Care Outcome Scale (Cicely Saunders Institute, 2012) websites.

2 Veronica's story was first published in our book *Life to Be Lived: Challenges and Choices for Patients and Carers in Life-Threatening Illnesses* (Proot & Yorke, 2014, p. 127).

3 Joanne was a Jungian therapist and used a sand tray in which Veronica could express her feelings with different materials.

References

Bruera, E., Higginson, I., von Gunten, C. & Morita, T., 2015. *Textbook of Palliative Medicine and Supportive Care*. 2nd edition. Abingdon: Taylor and Francis.

Carlson, C., 2016. Effectiveness of the World Health Organization Cancer Pain Relief Guidelines: An Integrative Review. *Journal of Pain Research*, Volume 9, pp. 515–534.

Cicely Saunders Institute, 2012. *Palliative Care Outcome Scale: A Resource for Palliative Care*. [Online] Available at: https://pos-pal.org [Accessed 3 November 2018].

Fitch, M. & Bartlett, R., 2019. Patient Perspectives About Spirituality and Spiritual Care. *Asia-Pacific Journal of Oncology Nursing*, Volume 6, pp. 111–121.

Giacino, J. & White, J., 2005. The Vegetative and Minimally Conscious States: Current Knowledge and Remaining Questions. *The Journal of Head Trauma Rehabilitation*, Volume 20, pp. 30–50.

Hatamipour, K., Rassouli, M., Yaghmaie, F., Zendedel, K. & Alavi Majd, H., 2015. Spiritual Needs of Cancer Patients: A Qualitative Study. *Indian Journal of Palliative Care*, Volume 21 (1), pp. 61–67.

McCullagh, P., 2004. *Conscious in a Vegetative State? A Critique of the PVS Concept*. Dordrecht: Kluwer Academic Publishers.

Mearns, D. & Cooper, M., 2005. *Working at Relational Depth in Counselling and Psychotherapy*. London: Sage Publications

Proot, C. & Yorke, M., 2014. *Life to Be Lived: Challenges and Choices for Patients and Carers in Life-threatening Illnesses*. Oxford: Oxford University Press.

Puchalski, C. et al., 2009. Improving the Quality of Spiritual Care as a Dimension of Palliative Care: The Report of the Consensus Conference. *Journal of Palliative Medicine*, Volume 12 (10), pp. 885–904.

Saunders, C., 1964. The Symptomatic Treatment of Incurable Malignant Disease. *Prescribers' Journal*, Volume 4 (4), pp. 68–73.

Seymour, J. & Clark, D., 2018. The Liverpool Care Pathway for the Dying Patient: A Critical Analysis of Its Rise, Demise and Legacy in England. *Wellcome Open Research*, Volume 3 (15).

Stroebe, M. & Shut, H., 1999. The Dual Process Model of Coping With Bereavement: Rationale and Description. *Death Studies*, Volume 23 (3), pp. 197–224.

The University of Edinburgh, 2010. *Supportive and Palliative Care Indicators Tool*. [Online] Available at: www.spict.org.uk [Accessed 17 January 2020].

World Health Organization, 2018. *WHOQOL: Measuring Quality of Life*. [Online] Available at: www.who.int/healthinfo/survey/whoqol-qualityoflife/en [Accessed 3 November 2018].

Chapter 2

The end of life – people's experiences

Having looked at beliefs and attitudes, we would now like to recall some experiences people have had towards the end of their life. The following story, introduced by one of his friends, pictures Alan sharing his experience when he was taken ill with a stroke and took a very long time to regain consciousness and some capacity. It gives a moving insight into the mystery of what patients and their loved ones can live through in the twilight of life.

Alan was a married and successful businessman of 60 years of age. One day he felt off colour, and this feeling continued for several days, but life continued normally as he enjoyed his new freedom as a retired person. Although he did not feel very well, he and his wife decided to accept a dinner invitation with friends. As the evening progressed, Alan began to feel ill, giddy and very cold. They decided it would be best to leave the party. That was just as well, because Alan was unable to drive home and could barely walk to his front door when they arrived. His wife called an ambulance because she noticed at that point that his face had dropped on one side, and she knew it could be a symptom of a stroke.

During the night in hospital, Alan had a seizure. In the early morning Alan's wife asked a friend if he would take her to the hospital, as she felt unable to drive. Both of them were shocked when they saw Alan. He looked as if he was dead, with no colour in his skin and hardly any sign of breathing. They experienced the suddenness and severity of the illness to be frightening.

Alan, for himself, later told of his total lack of any recognition of what was happening, until, in his words, he came to and was in a deep dream state. People came and went; he felt he was being rolled about on the floor; there were many strange noises and distant voices. "I felt like a child in a cot – I had no idea what was happening or who or what I was" Alan told us later. Eventually he became more aware of his surroundings and also the capacities he had lost. He could not speak or move some of his limbs. "I felt I was a sort of dummy, but at least there was no more pain!"

For his wife and family, this period was an absolute nightmare. They had no idea what was to happen or how they would cope with it. We listeners to this story realised again how a family can be hit by a desperate situation, which can affect their love for one another and their future. The questions came quickly and urgently. We observers could soon understand how a family can be the patient as well as the person in the bed.

The subsequent weeks and months were very difficult for Alan and his wife. They put great strains on their relationship and on his personal control through his frustration and anger at what he called the destruction of his retirement. It took a couple of years to gain some understanding and order, but the loss of much of his capacity to speak and move has confirmed his permanent predicament.

We write about the quality of life. That can, in some circumstances, become a dream hope, but life is still to be lived.

Alan's story speaks very movingly about the feelings and sensations that patients find themselves thrown into at the twilight of life. The story is tragic for one couple and family. How they managed and continue to do so raises powerful questions for them. When we are fit and well, it can be difficult for us to imagine what it is like to be struck down suddenly by serious or even potentially terminal illness. Alan's story articulates the shock, hopes and fears of family and friends. In what follows, we will describe more fully these feelings and other experiences at the twilight of life.

Patient experiences: a mixed bag of feelings and ordeals

Alan's story reveals something of the shock of sudden illness and the infliction on a person of quite new feelings and experiences. They can be traumatic for all those around the patient, especially the family. The patient himself needs to recognise that he has to accept a radically new and possibly stressful situation. That is very difficult if one does not feel well – very difficult to look down the future road of life and how long it is.

The same surrender needs to occur when the onset of the illness is slow and almost secret. Patients wonder why they cannot do the things which were natural and easy for them, even in the recent past. Sometimes it may be difficult to admit that one is ill, or one can feel embarrassed, not wanting to be different and coping perhaps with a reduction in personal control over one's life. As people get older, some of the symptoms seem natural, as they are associated with ageing. Sometimes people feel exposed by forgetfulness, weakness, deafness and their need for the toilet.

As things get worse, the process begins to frighten people. "How is this going to end? Am I going to die? Am I going to have acute pain? Does it mean hospital, surgery, medication?" Sometimes a fear develops about doctors, because they tell you bad news. Other people may look at doctors as saviours and even magicians. The questions keep coming – "Who can I trust? Is there hope of recovery to return to normal life?"

Such questions and many more like them can make the patient feel confused and uncertain about the future. The future itself is full of unknown facets, and these can frighten. Patients feel they have no strength or no willpower to cope. Frequently people going through such experiences become depressed. They do not know what is really happening and how they will cope. They may feel guilty about having to stop working or helping in the home and becoming increasingly reliant on other people. Fearing for the future, they may well dread what needs to be done before they die.

In the past, it was common that patients were not told of the nature of their illness or its consequences. Fortunately, today, that situation is rare but, sadly, not totally unknown. Furthermore, the bad news sometimes is broken very insensitively or vaguely, with the result that the patient may misunderstand the situation. They may become overwhelmed by it or even try to deny it. It is for them a new trauma, and their reaction can be both a physical and a psychological one.

Patients feel they have become an object and not a proper person; a passenger and not a driver. A sense of uselessness may grow and become pervasive. Their capacities seem to be curtailed in so many ways. At times like this, people may become short tempered. They change, and not always for the better. With growing weakness can come new feelings of shame, anger, fear, sadness and depression on top of the shock, pain and anxiety about their diagnosis and outlook. Death can become an escape, a subject of hope in the unknown and a sign of peace at not being a burden to oneself anymore or having to inflict it on others who care.

Being very ill and dying is not much fun; but when one is cared for appropriately, loved and understood, the sort of feelings recounted above can be put into a proper context. Hope may return; a positive view of the future, however potentially short, may be possible. The patient has to learn to hold on to the truth: "There are no certainties in medicine, only likelihoods. There are no certainties other than that all of us, at some time, will die". The timing of that event remains unclear, and perhaps it is just as well.

Loss

At the twilight of life, loss comes in many guises. There is the loss of connection with family, friends, work and society as a whole. But loss does not always involve other people. There is also a sense of a loss of power, authority, strength, control . . . all these things perhaps as a result of just simply getting frail. There is no escape from them. One has to accept it. There is a degree of acceptance which makes loss of capacity just about tolerable, yet, as we considered in our previous book, acceptance is never a given (Proot & Yorke, 2014, pp. 139–141). One can accept certain things, not others; one can experience acceptance one day and be void of any acceptance the next. The sense of loss is such a widespread thing that we all experience it even as we get older. In fact, we are dying all the time and losses become part of it.

In *How to Die: Simon's Choice* (2016), a BBC programme[1] first shown in February 2016, Simon's losses are very vividly depicted. He has to give up driving, let go of motivating his employees and eventually hand over his business altogether, thus getting disconnected from a society in which he can no longer be productive.

> The first time Simon fell over the dog, he was very upset. He realises the clock is ticking and says, "I'm independent. Like a used car, I'm worn out and it's not worth investing in repair". He experienced humiliation and helplessness and found it 'unmanly' to have a care worker help him shower and dress even if he recognises: "the person is so lovely that she lessens the blow".
>
> Simon's frustration at not being able to communicate is overwhelming, as he speaks four languages fluently. Trying to help his communication, he chooses a synthetic voice that can say what he writes on the computer. The perspective that, with his speech failing, his grandson will no longer understand him, and he would not be able to interact with him, brings him to say, "That barrier is SO terrible".
>
> And later he says: "I am terrified. I will lose my hand soon. My only form of interaction will be gone. No interaction is terrible". By contrast, when he sees the second doctor who comes to assess him on the eve of the procedure, he says, "I am zero % scared. It will be a relief. There is no fear to die".

The programme shows how difficult it was for Simon to adjust to the losses he was coming up against. Because of that, he was so set about going to Switzerland for assisted dying that nothing was going to change his mind; he was not prepared to look at anything else. Simon's attitude is an example of what a professor in palliative care we interviewed called 'the autonomy and the tunnel vision' by which he means that a patient sees autonomy as the ultimate or sole expression of their dignity, and when their independence is being eroded, they cannot come to terms with it. They say "I see only one possibility and that is it". It can also be a matter of getting absolute control. Sometimes, when people are in crisis, the possibility of euthanasia or assisted dying is the extreme control option, to gain or reclaim mastery over their life or death.

Trauma

Post-traumatic stress disorder (PTSD), while very real for the sufferers, remained unrecognised for what it was, and it was not until the Vietnam War that something of the true essence of PTSD was understood. In short, it is the traumatic experience of a person which is so awful that the memory of it is lodged deep in the subconscious so that, in effect, it can never be experienced again. The subconscious becomes a sort of protective shield. If the shield is damaged or broken, it can lead to symptoms appearing as aberrations, which can affect many parts of the body, mind and spirit. No part is safe. It is the range of presentations which can make diagnosis so difficult and lead to doctors and therapists being deceived as to what they are actually dealing with.

One of our consultants, Leslie, raised with us the importance of trauma at the end of life. Working in palliative care, he began to realise how often trauma was still not recognised by the medical profession. He asked eight of his colleagues how often they had met trauma in their day-to-day work. Some claimed some small experience, but only one had ever worked with it. In a small piece of research, using the strictest DSM-5[2] criteria, Leslie discovered that 30% of his bereaved clients had PTSD, and some of them had long-term developmental trauma. This confirms how important it is that trauma and PTSD are recognised and worked with seriously at the end of life.

A younger and healthier person who has suffered a traumatic experience can, with some effect, manage the physical and psychological assaults which cause them fears. The memory which is committed to the deep subconscious is held successfully by iron gates and heavy padlocks. The conscious mind can spend a lifetime keeping that memory locked up and 'safe'. As people get weaker, their defences against such assaults dwindle, and therefore the gates are forced open, and something of the force of the terrifying memory returns, raising great anxiety in the frailer person. The old trauma clearly still has its teeth. As the person begins the process of dying, their peace is disturbed, and the fears and stresses return. Such was the experience of Elaine.

> A woman in her forties, Elaine, seemed unable to die in spite of multiple organ failure. A psychologist noted the facts of her life and realised that she felt strongly that she had had a negative influence on her family and especially against her husband moving to higher office in his work. Elaine suffered profound subconscious guilt about this. The impact came as an addition to her fatal illness. The psychologist, after much thought and using his considerable experience, closed her subconscious negativity and she died peacefully four hours later.

When a trauma or something too painful occurs, our survival instinct puts a strategy into place to protect us from that ever happening again.

Unfortunately, in doing so, it also prevents us going anywhere near the traumatic memory. Many dying people have been trapped for years in such a complex which, though it helped them survive childhood abuse or trauma, did so at great personal cost. Sometimes their distress as they are dying is so great that their defences crumble and they can no longer contain their childhood pain, which bursts through. The following story, told by a palliative care physician, is an example.

> An elderly woman, Beth, became very upset on a hospice ward where I was working. When the nurses talked to her they discovered that she had had an illegitimate baby when she was only 15 years old. This had stayed with her, like a cancer gnawing at her mind, all through her life. She came from a working-class family where such an event was considered deeply shameful. The baby was adopted. She had never talked to anybody about it. As Beth lay dying, her defences broke down, and she collapsed in tears, unable to cope with her self-imposed silence anymore.

In a sense this was a profoundly healing moment for Beth when she was able to give voice to her shame in a climate of loving acceptance; how much more beneficial for her could it have been to exorcise the pain when she was younger?

This other story, told by Leslie, depicts how unresolved trauma can surface even more acutely at the twilight of life:

> An old white-haired Polish man, Janacek, was admitted to the ward with advanced cancer. He had a very heavy Polish accent, and he looked very pale and unwell. He was a quiet man, but after a few days he became confused, and as he talked, we realised he had become psychotic; he thought he was back in the concentration camp where he had been imprisoned during the war. Janacek thought that the doctors and nurses were guards and the other patients were his fellow inmates.
>
> Once, Janacek walked past a room where there was a person who had died. When he saw this his distress and confusion increased, as it reminded him of the many dead prisoners he had seen in the camp. At the time, all we could do was reduce his agitation with tranquillising medication. Sadly, we did not have a magic cure for him, but it was still a mercy to ease his anguish, to help him find a measure of calmness.

The memory of what had happened to Janacek stayed with Leslie, who realised later that a severe case of PTSD had overwhelmed Janacek's sanity at the end of his life. Somehow, Janacek had carried it for 30 years, but, weakened by his terminal illness, his defences could not cope anymore, and he fell back into his awful memories as if into a nightmare or trance state. If he had known then what he knew now, Leslie would have tried to find ways to help

Janacek to reconnect with reality, of helping him feel safe again, because he was so frightened. Janacek did not have long to live, so prolonged therapy was not going to be possible. It would have to be measures like someone sitting with him whenever he felt anxious and emphasising an empathic connection with Janacek.

It is powerfully clear that supportive human presence is needed in crises. One could be looking to find ways of making physical contact if the patient felt safe enough to accept that, maybe simply by holding their hand. We have a deep primal need rooted in early childhood to be held, touched, stroked and rocked to soothe us. We would want to teach the staff about reading a patient's body as much as hearing their words, watching out for fast breathing, a raised pulse rate, pale skin in a cold sweat, a dry mouth, restless movements . . . all signs of stress and distress.

It is really important to recognise these cues and to be knowledgeable about this, looking for anything which re-establishes human contact, trying to find an anchor which will bring the patient back to reality instead of being caught in a hellish state. In what he calls 'pre-therapy', Gary Prouty (Prouty, 1994; Van Werde & Morton, 1999) suggests the use of reflections focussing on the here and now, the moods and the relationship, to help severely disturbed patients reconnect with reality. This clearly conveys that beyond the provision of drugs and symptom control, there is the vital 'presence', which is what Dame Cicely Saunders affirmed in her repeated use of the phrase 'watch with me', which became the title of one of her books (2003).

Trauma affects the body, mind, emotions, relationships and spirit. Its treatment needs a holistic approach. In trauma therapies, when people recover from PTSD, there is a phenomenon called post-traumatic growth whereby that healed person comes back to life, rediscovers the life in themselves, and taps into sources of creativity and resilience they never knew they had. This discovery is profoundly hopeful. Charles, a Jungian therapist, spoke of Ella.[3]

Ella was the wife of a distinguished army officer who had hitherto filled her life with travel and making and meeting many artist friends. These relationships stimulated her, but as she grew older, arthritis began to restrict her movements, and Ella gradually became isolated and lonely.

At a low time, Ella met Charles and regaled him with her stories, and as a result of her memories, she lost some of her fear of death. She developed a new meaning to her life. She was not going to be a hero like her husband or famous like some of her friends; she found and accepted her own place in life, however modest that may be.

A few years later Charles received a call saying Ella was very ill in hospital. They had heard her using Charles's name and assumed she wanted to see him. Ella had been in a coma and hadn't spoken, eaten or drunk. Charles went. He remembers, "She was just lying there, in a room on her own. I was sitting at her bedside, quietly meditating. Suddenly, she sat up, bolt upright, opened her eyes, looked at me and said, "You've come. I just wanted to say thank you". We both cried, she lay down, I left and she died.

That she seems to have come out of her coma to thank Charles is incredibly moving. Ella's story is a striking example of how a life's journey can tend towards completion and fulfilment despite and through limiting circumstances. We have heard many stories of people reaching such a place and crossing that last river peacefully. Some dying people are open and ready to do this; some are too ill; some are not ready.

Surely it is the role of the carer of any sort, if possible, to help the dying people to move towards this as best they can. How can they do that? A multidisciplinary team working holistically enables each discipline to provide their unique skills – medical, nursing, social work, physiotherapy, massage, acupuncture, chaplaincy and more. A skilled psychotherapist is needed, too, who understands trauma and how to work with the body as well as family members or close friends who know how to be supportive. We have only begun to develop the skills needed to support people who have been traumatised. There is more to learn, particularly about the language of the body and that of the psyche, which, in ancient Greece, meant soul. In medicine, one may be diagnosed with a myocardial infarction; in the language of psyche you have a broken heart. Both can mend; one is perhaps more helpful to the non-medical patient.

Pain and suffering

It is important to differentiate not only the generality of suffering when someone is dying but also the difference between pain and suffering and their distinct source. We consider in general that pain is locatable and specifically identifiable in the mechanisms of the physical body: a broken leg, a cancer, muscle weakness, etc. Physical pain can take the form of an ache, nausea, weakness, breathlessness, hunger or thirst and also the humiliating symptoms of urinary and faecal incontinence. But the patient also responds to that experience of pain, and that we can call suffering; the loss of ability, a sense of isolation and lack of understanding, dependency and its stress on caregivers, etc. Pain is essentially physical; suffering is emotional, psychological, spiritual, environmental. The perception of physical pain and suffering can vary according to the circumstances. The same pain can be unbearable when one is alone in the middle of the night and be forgotten the next morning when meeting a friend.

Suffering is a more pervasive feeling that overwhelms or threatens the whole person, on their own behalf or that of somebody else who triggers their own feelings. Thus, if a person badly cuts themselves, they suffer pain in the place where they cut. The friend who is there can suffer in response to that person's pain and through their own feelings of pity, dread, anxiety . . . They can seek to help that person by noticing the pain and looking for a way to relieve it. Most of the time one can treat pain with painkillers, but even when the pain is reduced, the suffering may continue, because drugs do not have the same power over suffering as over pain.

Suffering may not only be a hazier version of pain, but it can also be long term and in the whole person as a weight of guilt, fear or lostness. It can become a matter of the soul, with strong connections with emotions. Joyce's suffering is an example of this:

> Joyce had killed her new-born baby because she could not take on the respon-
> sibility of motherhood. A diversionary factor which informed strongly some of
> the help offered to Joyce was that the baby was black, the product of a brief
> liaison outside her marriage.

Joyce's suffering was not physical, but the expression of her feelings was. The source of suffering is more located in the heart, but it is no less painful for that. We think, for example, of an inability to see a bright future, moodi-ness, recollection of the past, questioning the meaning of life and where we belong. The different sources of pain and suffering bring different reactions. Pain can be outshone by more powerful stimuli, and people can lift them-selves over pain, as we can see in the stories of Beatrix and Emma, which follow. Pain can also fill a gap caused by boredom and lack of external motivation.

One of the major problems in our culture is that we cannot cope with suffering anymore. This leads to the abusive use of anti-depressants and analgesic medication, which can bring serious limitations to our capacity to manage pain in the same way as the overuse of antibiotics makes them less effective when a body really needs their support to fight of an infec-tion. An interviewee, a chaplain in a university hospital, told us of his experience:

> Every week I come across situations we would regard as a very good way of
> dying, a normal process, without pain and anxiety; this mother or father or
> son is just slipping away into death. Yet the family surrounding the bed are
> saying "This is intolerable, this is not humane, this is not human dignity. DO
> something". And we have to respond, "No. This is the normal way people die.
> This is a good way to die".
>
> This happens when people cannot recognise that they are suffering
> because the other one is suffering. We have to detach our feelings of pain
> from the fact that we ache out of sympathy with the other one's suffering. If
> we are confused about the source of our pain, we do not recognise what is

happening, and we cannot really respond to the suffering of the other person. Unfortunately, such confusion is common in our culture, and people are thus unable to respond appropriately most of the time.

I have come across someone aged 70 saying that this was the first time that they had seen someone die. Somehow, such people are not acquainted with the processes of life and death, of living and dying. I think this is one of the reasons why many people say that if someone in end of life asks for euthanasia, they should be given it, and everything would be solved. The process of dying is frightening because it is unfamiliar, and I think often euthanasia is used as a way to run away from what is quite natural.

Although there is room for both the patient's suffering and for that of the bystander, we need to separate and distinguish what is our suffering from what is theirs. Doctors and nurses, as in Anthony's story, the young boy who wanted to remain as conscious as possible despite the pain, may see their inability to do something to relieve pain as a failure. They realise they cannot work their magic – they have their own suffering. Another example is that of a spouse of a terminal patient who is suffering at the thought of what is to come, the uncertainty of how long her ordeal will be and of her coming widowhood. Some will respond to this suffering by rejecting or denying it. But this lady also suffers for her husband's pain and loss of capacity, and unless she is able to differentiate the source of her ache and make the distinction between her pain and his pain, her suffering and his suffering, she will not be able to really listen to or hear what her husband is saying; she will not be able to be present and sit with him in his experiencing.

Sometimes patients who do not seem in excessive pain can feel huge suffering because of their mental attitude to it. A chaplain recounted the following story of Eugene.

> Eugene, a patient who was due to be euthanised, asked me to stay with him, and my last words to him were "You are very self-centred".
>
> Eugene had had backache for a year. His GP sent him to a physiotherapist, but that treatment did not improve matters. In the end, he sent the patient to have some scans, which revealed that he had full-blown cancer. Nothing could be done to cure him.
>
> Although Eugene's pain was not any worse than when he came in, when given the diagnosis, this man refused everything. He refused to go home, he would not read the paper, he would not watch television . . . the only thing he said was "I want euthanasia. If you can't cure me or treat me, you will have to kill me".
>
> When I met his wife, it transpired that she did not know anything about the running of the household. I told Eugene that he needed to inform her as he

was preparing to die. But whatever I said to him, he did not alter his stance. Eugene was not in intolerable pain. His suffering was psychological because he knew he was going to die, and that made it intolerable for him to go on living, so he wanted to die now.

So my last words to him were, "Why do you remain so selfish?!" Just before he was euthanised, his wife asked him something, and he did not even respond anymore. He was not in a terrible state, he could have responded, but he was closed up in himself. Perhaps that was who he was.

His wife came to see me regularly after his death, repeating time and again the same conversation: "Why couldn't he say the necessary things? Why couldn't he say goodbye? Even more, he made me angry, because I did not know what insurances we had".

As long as Eugene had a backache, he could cope with the pain. When it turned out to be cancer and his outlook became death rather than a cure, his suffering became unbearable, and he angrily locked everything and everybody out of his life. As the reader, we should be careful about making a judgement. To the outsider, this story and Eugene's attitude can seem very selfish and even aggressive. He did not care an iota about what happened after he left this world. He could not be in it any longer, so to hell with it. He would not overcome his (moral) pain nor do anything to help the people, even his wife, who would be alive and kicking when he would be dead. He could not care less.

As the story ends perhaps, this was who Eugene was, and he did not have the mental strength or the capacity to be any different. Even the chaplain could not break through the suffering Eugene was locked in. Eugene was unwilling to meet him and talk about the bigger picture. The only thing the chaplain could do was to keep supporting Eugene's wife for months after his death, because she was left with a very complicated grieving process because of his attitude. As someone told us, sometimes euthanasia solves a problem for the patient but at the same time creates another problem for those who are surviving them.

Unbearable pain or suffering

In the countries where there is legislation by which people are allowed to ask for euthanasia, one of the criteria is that the patient is in 'intolerable pain' that cannot be relieved. But what is intolerable pain? A physician told us:

For many people, intolerability is a concept about the future. They fear their illness, their pain, their suffering will become intolerable. Actually, they don't know. They are basing their view on others' experiences, which may not apply to them.

> Many patients have told me they don't want antibiotics if they get an infection; they just want to be allowed to die. But when they do get an infection and by chance they feel a little better, they change their minds and decide to have further treatment after all.

It is not that easy to define what 'intolerable pain' is. It will be different for every single person and, as this physician rightly comments, often based on fears and beliefs of others. Someone shared with us their fear of dying in words such as "I have seen my mother in such great pain, I do not want that to happen to me". What people fear or hope for cannot be taken for granted, and very often, when asked "Do you want the doctor to give you an injection to kill you?" which is what euthanasia is, they reply, "Oh no, but I don't want to be in pain".

We want to encourage caregivers and family members not to shy away from having a conversation about intolerable pain and not to take their expression of a death wish for granted. So much more can come to the fore if we take the time to look at the question behind the question, at the fear behind the statement. We might ask what exactly is intolerable? The fear of overwhelming pain or suffocation or other symptoms? Anxiety about treatments such as chemotherapy, with its high level of side-effects and horror stories they have heard from others? Not wanting to be vulnerable or disabled? A fear of becoming confused? These are not set in stone. The whole point of palliative care is that there are nearly always ways of relieving such symptoms.

Finding meaning

With Viktor Frankl's logotherapy (Frankl, 2004) and Cicely Saunders's concept of 'total pain' (Clark, 2014), the question of meaning has entered the world of medicine. Here follows the story of a conversation between a palliative care physician in a university hospital and a patient, exemplifying how relevant questions can make a difference in how patients value their life.

> Steven was a man of 65 with lung cancer. He was disappointed about his life. I was doing my daily round of the patients, and he was sitting there. He was not satisfied, and I asked him what was happening. He said that he was just reflecting about his life, which had not been successful. I sat down and asked whether I could do something for him.
>
> He then told me that he had divorced 15 years previously and that his ex-wife came to visit him the day before with their two sons. He said that it did not do anything for him whether she was there or not and that he did not want her to come back. After 15 years, there was no way that she could appear on the announcement of his death. And it would be impossible that she could be at the funeral. He was angry.

I said that I realised he was disappointed about his marriage and proceeded to ask about his work. He replied that he had been employed for his whole career in the same manufacturing company, and it was fine. So I said that was good. I also said that I had noticed his two sons were visiting him every day on the palliative care unit, so it seemed to me that he had a very close relationship with his children. He agreed, and he was very proud of them. They had a diploma and were employed, and each had a good wife, and his grandchildren came in to see him.

I remarked to him that I saw that he was a normal man. I also suggested that if I was asking a student in an examination three questions and they answered as he did, I would give the students a mark of two and a half for positivity. That had to be very good.

He looked at me, puzzled. Two and a half? he asked. I said that his employment record was good; secondly, that his relationship with his children seemed fine; and it was just his marriage that after 15 years featured a divorce. So, two and a half of the three very important things in his life were excellent. I continued that I did not know anybody who was perfect, not even myself. He looked at me, and I told him to think about it all.

The next day he told me that he had been thinking about what I had said and that maybe I was right. He maintained that his wife was not to appear in the funeral announcement. I then asked him if he could imagine what his sons would feel losing their dad while still having a good relationship with their mum. Was it possible that they might have some support from their mum at that difficult time?

He realised that he had not looked at it this way. I suggested that he might discuss it with his boys and then maybe leave the final decision to them as to what they wanted to do. They would have to decide whether or not they needed the support of their mother when they were saying goodbye to their father. He obviously continued to think about it, and four days later he told me that they had to do what they thought was good.

It was as if in spite of all the anger and the reflection about his wife, he could move to a totally different conclusion, realising that he could still do things for his sons to enable them to say afterwards, "We had a good dad, and at the end of his life, he became mild, and he could see what he could do for us by not blocking off the support of our mum". Maybe in this way it was very useful that he was able to discuss this with his sons and to overcome his wariness about his wife while giving support to the boys.

Steven's story shows that the issues he was dealing with were not just a medical problem, but they were social, existential and psychological. The relevant questions to help people give meaning to their experience at the twilight of life are:

- What can I do?
- What is my life?
- How do I look back on my life? and
- Looking forward, how can I do something? How can I make a difference?

That is real palliative and terminal care: it is about how we guide patients so that they become satisfied with their experience. Finally, this patient, instead of being disappointed about his life, was satisfied that even in his terminal situation, he could do something that was important for his sons and also for his daughters-in-law and grandchildren – and maybe his wife too. So they could become unified. A connection was made which gave licence to the fact that they were connected and which was recognised and important.

Lifting oneself over pain

Eugene, although 'objectively' in no more pain than he was before the cancer diagnosis, saw his suffering multiplied by the terminal outlook, and he could see nothing else. He was locked in his suffering. The following story of Emma shows a different experience. Her pain could not easily be controlled, and yet she found ways to lift herself over the pain, if only for that special day. Her palliative care physician tells her story.

> Emma was young, very good looking. She had breast cancer with bone secondaries, which produced severe pain. It was a struggle all the time to try and find a way to control her pain. During her final illness, she decided to get married. She had a partner and a child.
>
> What was so striking was how they lived the whole ceremony. She bought a silk wedding dress, and the nurses helped her to get ready. It was a special ritual, like any other woman preparing for marriage, and yet unlike. Theirs was a proper ceremony, not just a few words at the bedside; she really went for it.
>
> I knew that she was in severe pain, but you actually couldn't tell. She looked well, she was determined to have her day, and she did. Somehow, she managed to lift herself above her pain for the day.

Marriages happen in the hospice, much to people's surprise. They may not be familiar with the hospice ideal and how they are places of living more than of dying. Such marriages are testimony to how people can lift themselves, with the help of others often, over the pain and suffering, which no longer define who they are. People are much more than their pain, and although this is difficult, as pain tends to overwhelm and take all the space, it is good to know and believe that it can be reduced to just part of one's experience, often by strengthening or developing another or new parts of who they are.

Thus, it happened in a hospice where a nurse had heard some breast cancer patients talking amongst themselves about their body image and how hard it was to go to a shop and buy a dress. It spurred the care team to contact a designer school and invite them round for a project, helping each lady design and make their own dress. The project culminated in a catwalk on which each lady exhibited their dress. The smiles on their faces; the confidence and the pleasure they got out of the whole project were stunning. For a while they could feel normal, even special, and were not limited to their pain and suffering. One of them, an African lady, chose to design her wedding dress, a beautiful orange dress with special matching headscarf, and chose to be buried in that dress (Hartley et al., 2010).

Remission

As we have noted before, there are no certainties in medicine; it is always a matter of probability. Medicine is not an exact science, and time and again, professionals are confronted with the uncertainty and unpredictability of their trials and errors, which, for the patient and the family who are desperate to 'know', can be very difficult to live with. How often have we heard patients saying "Even bad news would be better than living with the not knowing?" But unpredictability can also surprise us in a positive way as the following story of a palliative care physician tells us.

> I went to see a woman, call her Linda, who was referred to me with terminal liver cancer. A third of her abdomen was filled with the liver tumour. She had lung secondaries, the chest X-ray showing multiple round lesions. I went to see Linda at home. What I expected was someone very ill, thin and bedbound. I rang the doorbell, and a woman opened the door. She looked well, normal. I asked if I could see the patient and she said, "Oh, that's me". I was somewhat surprised!
>
> When I went through her history, she told me she had no symptoms, had plenty of energy, and everything was fine. When I examined her, I found that her previously hugely enlarged liver had somehow almost disappeared, having shrunk down to normal size.
>
> I thought, 'There is something odd going on here', so I sent her back for investigation. The chest X-ray showed that her lung secondaries had gone, and ultrasound indicated that the liver had indeed shrunk right down. A repeat biopsy simply showed fibrous tissue. She was in spontaneous remission from advanced cancer despite not having had any treatment.
>
> Linda was OK with her remission. She really did not want to talk about it much, but she had a very strong faith and she did say there was a moment

when she knew it was going to be all right. She didn't say any more, so I thought that there was much more happening here that she did not want to go into. It was important to respect her privacy, even if it left one with a sense of loss as to cause and effect.

This story shows that the seemingly impossible does happen in medicine. Even in hospices, where patients are all supposed to be imminently dying, you sometimes see people who survive much longer than their progress indicates. This experience taught that physician that our understanding of the healing process is still very limited. It is not that spontaneous remissions happen often. They do not; they are rare. Nevertheless, in PubMed, the American database of medical publications, lists, on average, four case reports a month of spontaneous remissions from cancer are recorded.

We came across a doctor who said he could tell whether someone would live or die. "I sort of smell it", he said. He suggested that a core of survival is whether the patient is genuinely happy or not. More generally, there is a lot of interest now in whether a person's state of mind, a strong belief that they will get better and a determination to do so, may affect their outcome. Sophie Sabbage, the writer of *The Cancer Whisperer* (Sabbage, 2016), who had advanced lung cancer with multiple metastases, is an example. She showed extraordinary determination in her pursuit of a healing process, which she remained in charge of, combining orthodox medical and unorthodox complementary therapies, which led to her metastases disappearing and her original tumour shrinking. In theory, this should not have happened. How people respond to their illness, however serious, may in some cases affect the outcome.

Carers' experiences: sharing or mirroring the patient's

So far, we have focused on the patient's experience, but family and carers suffer too. Watching a loved one suffer, noticing their disease progression and the dwindling of their strength and capacity and feeling helpless to do anything about it, can be very taxing for the next of kin. Intimate relationships are exposed when one can no longer show affection in the usual way. And as we discussed in our earlier book (Proot & Yorke, 2014), partners and family take on a number of new roles such as being a carer and spokesperson with the medical team, whilst they also juggle with the old ones of both partners in the family routine of meals, school runs, bins, banking and admin. No wonder they suffer huge fatigue, and there is little or no time to pay attention to their own feelings, which cones at a cost.

For the medical team, terminal illness of a patient is difficult too. Trained to cure and treat, they feel they fall short. Being with a very ill patient and accepting that there is nothing one can do therapeutically to help is very painful for the physician. The temptation to seek refuge in more, even unnecessary treatment is real. It is never easy to move from the position of a physician who acts and prescribes to the one who can only listen and be present, especially in situations of prolonged distress.

Sometimes, patient and family members have similar or mirrored experiences. They may want to protect each other and pretend all is well; they may agonise each in their own corner about the situation, their fears, fantasies and hopes; they may also find support in each other's acceptance of their ordeal and deepen their relationship in the twilight of their life together. In what follows, different stories highlight some of these shared and/or mirrored experiences.

Protection of self and others

We referred earlier to the BBC programme featuring Simon, a MND patient, in the nine months leading up to his voluntary death in Switzerland (*How to Die: Simon's Choice*, 2016). In this programme, the interactions between Simon and his friends and family members and how they impact on their relationship are poignantly described.

> Simon's wife is against assisted dying, and she does not want to go to Switzerland with him. When, suddenly, the prospect is in her face, she is "utterly terrified of what it will be like". She is also frightened to upset Simon any more by trying to persuade him not to do it. So she tries to avoid the conversation and make everyday life okay. She cannot talk about his plan because, she says, "it makes it more real". Yet a family friend comments, "Simon is very forceful. If she was more resolute it would be more difficult for him".
>
> A few weeks later Simon attempts suicide, which somehow turns his wife round. Because of her fears and hesitation and her lack of outright support for his Switzerland project, she feels responsible for Simon's suicide attempt. She writes in an invitation to the farewell party they are organising for Simon. "In light of the recent developments, Switzerland is the kindest and best option considering one hell of a week we have had. Please know that you will find us beaten, battle-weary, bruised and broken". To a certain extent, a friend thinks along similar lines when he says "Simon's suicide attempt demonstrates the depth of his distress". In the face of the suicide attempt, the focus is Simon's distress; their feelings are second best.
>
> Simon's mother recognises this is a big step to take. Simon is still taking part in things, he can still write, and he is getting so much support from everybody. Her stance is to respect his choice, yet in doing so, her own preferences are excluded. "I won't encourage him, but I will go with whatever he wants. We both cried when we said goodbye, which he did not want. He did not invite

me to Switzerland, but I was looking forward to going. It was my son. I cannot get another son. He was brave. I don't have the option of being brave or not".

Friends are feeling distraught. A friend has cried every time he has seen Simon for the last two months. They are crushed that he has chosen a date to kill himself, and a friend warns Simon, "Your wife has rights in this. She has doubts".

The film, unfortunately, does not relay what Simon's reaction was to this email, and we could not help but be surprised at how little empathy Simon shows to his mother, his friends or his wife. When the latter expresses her doubts about him going to Switzerland, he says, "Her fright causes me sadness" and does not even seem aware of his wife's sadness and pain. This may be an example of how in time of illness, the patient's whole world contracts, and there can be a degree of self-centredness. Michael Mayne describes very clearly, in *The Enduring Melody*, how his concerns centred around the illness and his body changes. His sleep was affected by the anticipation and anxiety which crept up on him in the dark hours of the night. Such feelings made him more self-centred and aware and, he tells us, "self-concern is a near neighbour of self-indulgence" (Mayne, 2006, p. XIX).

A Macmillan nurse, call her Leila, reminded us that, sometimes, being around people who are dying can be unbearable, even for the professional. Mostly it is bearable because the patient is not their family, but it has happened that she connected with the awfulness of what was happening too much for her own protection. She recalls:

I can remember a young couple. Tim was about 40 years old, and with Jane, they had two small boys. On one visit, I found Tim desperately ill, on oxygen and struggling to breathe, and Jane was feeding him raw beetroot and salad leaves because she said, "This is what is going to get him better". I can remember visiting again when he was actually dying, when he was clearly in the last hours, I could not bear observing the scene and her obvious agony at the bedside.

This was very difficult for Leila, but she says mostly she manages, because of her own level of acceptance of death and dying. She loves the phrase 'Nature taking its course' and feels other people find that a helpful way of viewing things too sometimes.

When it is your own family, Leila admits, it makes it that much harder. It can be very difficult being the child but with some understanding of the situation and a sense of responsibility to be the nurse for the family too, as when her mother would phone her in a great deal of pain, asking, "What do I do? What do I do?" and she would talk her through taking a dose of her morphine. Leila has been in the position of health professional and family member three times. But she believes personal loss has made her better at her job. It has enabled her to do it differently, through her own understanding and insight, she hopes. She feels the emotion hugely for people, but she manages it. She believes that if professionals cannot do this, they have to stop doing such work. Leila remembers:

> After mum had died, I was working in a cancer ward. My mother's death made my job, on occasions, really difficult. I was going to visit a woman to break the bad news to her regarding her own diagnosis. She was in a bed upstairs on one of the top floors in the hospital, and all I could see as I sat with her was the image of my mother in that bed. Then I knew it was time to stop and have a change, and that is when I went back to palliative care.

Leila's testimony reminds us that professional carers are human beings with feelings and emotions and that the work they are doing touches them. This is why supervision, creativity and other ways of helping professionals deal with their feelings, compassion fatigue and vicarious trauma are so important. And as Leila so bravely states, at times, their personal and professional lives can become entangled, but working through it can make them better professionals. Many readers may have heard stories along the lines of this heart surgeon friend who, after having been a patient in hospital himself, fundamentally changed the way he talked and dealt with patients.

Thus, protection of self and others can take many guises. Sometimes all one can do is blind oneself to the other's pain and/or to our own pain, pretending everything is well. Unfortunately, this often stands in the way of open communication and sharing, and people tend to become estranged from each other. We remember discussing such an attitude with a patient's husband who was caring for her 24/7, enveloping her in cotton wool. Recognising the rift that was widening between them, he could give himself permission to become her husband again, lying beside each other on the bed when she was resting and sharing their hopes and fears. There are no rights and wrongs at the twilight of life. Everybody is doing the best they can, whether they are family or professional, and when they can acknowledge how they could try things differently and act upon it, the relationship and the quality of interaction can be improved.

What will happen next?

Whether after a long illness or due to the shock of sudden illness, patients and people around them hardly ever feel they are prepared for what is happening to them. One of our interviewees had the following story:

> My friend Richard had a serious stroke which left him initially in a flattened vegetative state. I questioned, "What is the future for him and his good

wife? Does he understand the situation?" In the early stages, he looked utterly miserable. If his mind was working, and one does not know about that, he looked to be saying, "How on earth has this happened to me and why? Will it ever end?" He looked deeply frustrated by the condition he was in. Possibly his mind was working, but he was totally incapable of expressing himself.

Richard's condition was very challenging for his friend. It caused him to think about the unpreparedness of everybody around him to answer clearly the question when Richard was so ill: 'Can and should his life be brought to a quiet close?' Precious little help to tackle that question seemed to be available to him or anybody in his circle, which left Richard wondering in confusion and isolation.

In the story of Peter, the father of two young boys who wanted to die on his sofa, both the nurse and the GP took a lot of time to explain what might happen – but not only to explain, also to prepare for what might be happening. The GP told us:

> I think in palliative care it is very important to foresee things, to prepare people for what is coming, so that when the time comes – and dying is not always so beautiful (sometimes it is but sometimes it isn't) – people can understand what is happening. When people know what to expect, I feel it makes it more bearable for them.
>
> It is important to recognise – even in a situation where you have the impression that it is understood by everybody – that the tempo, the speed and clarity of understanding can be different for people. They have a general feeling about what is about to happen, but they have also a personal feeling, and both are not always in balance. Therefore, it is very important once in a while or quite frequently to ask them "How is it for you now?" As a GP, we are not only focussed on the patient; it is important to remember that the family is the patient too.

It was beautiful to see the humanity of this GP, who could empathise with what it is like for the patient and their family who, even when they have been told, may not have fully understood what is to occur next nor what they might expect. His awareness and sensitivity to what makes death and dying more bearable for the patient and his family is obvious when he goes the extra mile in asking repeatedly how things are for them in this moment and in repeating what they might expect to happen next.

A palliative care physician commented on how staff can sometimes whinge, "This is a difficult person. This is a crazy family". His immediate answer to such statement is: "Yes, they are difficult because they are in a difficult situation. They have never learned how to handle such a threat before.

They are not experienced". As professional caregivers, we have to understand that this situation is difficult for them, and that is why they behave in a difficult way. There is a crisis, and they behave in the crisis, and we need to avoid going into crisis too. Instead, we have to try and understand why it is so difficult for them. A conversation could take place as follows:

- What makes this situation so difficult for you? Were you not prepared that the disease was so serious?
- No, never. Nobody told us.
- Oh, let's sit down and look at what we can do now or what we can't do. Have all alternative treatments been used? Is there an option left? Is it worth trying, yes or no? Would you like to try it? Do you want to try it for yourself?

In this physician's experience, many patients say, "I don't want to be treated anymore, but my children are pushing me". Or "My partner is pushing me because they are not ready to lose me". He feels the doctor can explore with the patient and the family whether they have the right to push their partner or a family member to go through a treatment to which they have objections. What rule gives them or denies them the right to interfere? Doctors can help patient and family see as clearly as possible what the process is and why they are doing or not doing something. It can be a useful way of bridging the gap to what will happen next.

Hope and courage

Hope is a 'virtue' in Christian theological terms, a combination of the desire for something and the expectation of receiving it. Hope may be vague – things will get better – or very specific – for safe return from a journey. In our experience, it is certainly very powerful yet utterly mysterious in its presence or absence and in the way in which it works. Courage, the resolve to act virtuously, especially when it is most difficult, is a gift that can spring from hope.

In the BBC programme *How to Die: Simon's Choice* (2016), it transpires that Simon's stepdaughter, who died of leukaemia two years previously, had asked her mother at one point to kill her. The palliative care team stepped in and sorted it out, and the following day, the daughter apologized, and they had a few more months of positive time.

> As her mum reflects on that experience, she wonders why this is different. With her daughter, there was still hope, and she wonders why Simon cannot feel that. Her husband's lack of hope makes her angry. She hates him feeling a burden and less worthy to be alive because of the illness. Yet she feels helpless to do anything about it.

Meanwhile, friends feel shocked that "Simon seems to be checking out before his time". They would like to stop the accelerating speed of change in his condition. They try to offer practical help in walking the dog. They are dreading the November date and cope by disbelieving it. "It's going so quickly". Simon's sister thinks he is still enjoying life: "He laughs so much" she says. She recognises that his wife doesn't want him to go but feels that in the end, it has to be his choice. "What is Simon going to be if he cannot communicate?" The games, she thinks, may be a way of Simon deflecting attention. And reflecting on the whole episode, she recognises, "He was brave, but we have to remember the people who have to sit it out and endure. They have to be brave too!"

Simon's wife experiences a range of conflicting feelings: she is furious, tender, loving, protective and says, "Simon has made it very clear he wants no more. It is terribly sad. If you love someone you have to do what they want to do. I am thankful that I met him". Two weeks after his death, she continues: "I remember the tenderness I had for Simon, preparing him the last morning, making him look smart as he liked it. I had to get through it for him. For him it was exactly the right time. For us it is extraordinarily difficult. I feel angry. I am missing him. I yearn. I feel guilty that I could not make his life nice enough". The gift of love can cause suffering but also pride, thankfulness and hope.

The range of patient and family responses to their ordeal never ceases to surprise us. An oncologist described his experience of how, although a patient may know they are unwell, it comes as a terrific surprise and shock when they are told that they are dying. We wonder if this could be something about instinctively being geared on survival even if they know that sometimes the illness and its symptoms can relapse. Or could it be that the shock comes because of a change from normality, in the sense that it may have become normal to be ill but not to die? Or else could it be something relational by which it is only when our being unwell is confirmed in someone's eyes or conversation that it sinks in?

We have more questions than answers, as we are reminded of a patient who had been asking his GP again and again, in the days when it was not usual to talk with patients about their diagnosis: "Do tell me that I have cancer. I know that I have. Do tell me". When eventually in the face of such insistence the GP broke the news, the patient encouraged him never to do so again. He said "As long as you had not said the word, I had hope. Now I know that it is terminal".

Hope and courage are mysterious and powerful ingredients at the twilight of life. How we manage or even spark them will be different for everyone but no less important if and when we can do something to keep these gifts alive. But sometimes, we cannot, and that helplessness and the deep solitude that come with it can be very hard to bear.

Curiosity and acceptance

If the way people are with their illness can in some cases affect the outcome, it also affects the quality of their life and that of the people around them. An oncologist told us the story of Beatrix, a patient who has stayed with him over the years, struck as he was by what transpired in her attitude.

> Beatrix, a woman of about 60, had ovarian cancer. She was an outpatient. I saw her on a regular basis. As we journeyed along, we always discussed the next treatment. She said, "Life is so beautiful for me. I want to take all of it". She wanted all the treatment she could have.
>
> When I had no more treatment to offer Beatrix, we talked about end of life. "I don't want to be sedated, I don't want euthanasia", she said. "Death belongs to life, and I want to live that part of life as well". It was very impressive. The way she said it was very strong. It stands out in my mind and memory! I have never experienced such an attitude before nor since.
>
> Beatrix was living very intensely. She enjoyed music, played a lot of music, and she had a full life. It was easy for the staff to deal with her. She was very clear in her expression. She did have her aches and pains but was dealing with them very easily. She was clear about them because she knew, she accepted, and still worked away at them. We had very clear conversations about end of life. I talked to her family, who told me she died very quietly.

What helped Beatrix in dealing with her aches and pains so easily may well have been her outlook on life: for her, positive and negative sides all belonged to life as a whole. Beatrix was curious about how it is to die; her attitude was positive. Most people have a negative attitude towards death and dying and are anxious. Some do not want to know. They want to avoid talking about it altogether. Others want to know as many details as possible; they want to control. This story shows that curiosity and acceptance can influence the way in which people die . . . and live as well.

Sometimes, unfinished business stands in the way of acceptance and letting go at the end of life. A palliative care physician tells the story of Alberto.

> I looked after a Mediterranean patient who was close to death. Alberto had become estranged from his daughter and son. When we found this out, we got the sense that he was hanging on in the hope of seeing them before he died.
>
> We went into a kind of overdrive to try to find these people. The Salvation Army, who are expert at this, helped and found his daughter first. She came in, and we could see a reconciliation taking place. We thought, "Ah, okay, this is it. Alberto can die now". But he still hung on.

Eventually we found his son, and he came in, and again they met and reconciled. A day or so later, Alberto was dead. He had resolved the alienation between him and his children. That was clearly crucially important to him and allowed him to die, I hope, peacefully.

Alberto's story shows that acceptance is something about wholeness and balance. There may always be bits that are not right, but when an overall sense of wholeness or completion is achieved or maintained, the patient can let go and die peacefully. This is helpful for the family, too, who, having settled unfinished business with their closest and dearest, can move on with their grieving, unburdened by guilt and regrets.

To go further. . .

1   Questions and experiences can make a patient feel confused at the end of life. What cues can help me assess which areas to focus on? How would I want to support them accordingly?
2   Can I give an example to explain whether and how physical pain and suffering can be different? How would I assess and address them as a carer?
3   Can I name three more common worries in people involved in end-of-life care? How can I make a difference as a professional?

Acknowledgements

Text extracts from Mayne, M., *The Enduring Melody*, Darton, Longman and Todd, London, UK, Copyright © 2006, reproduced with permission from Darton, Longman and Todd publishers.

Text extracts from Proot, C. & Yorke, M., *Life to Be Lived: Challenges and Choices for Patients and Carers in Life-threatening Illnesses*, Oxford University Press, Oxford, UK, Copyright © 2014, reproduced with permission of the Licensor through PLSclear.

Notes

1 The three-stage documentary follows Simon, an MND (motor neuron disease) patient, his family and friends, during nine months leading up to his voluntary death in Switzerland.
2 *Diagnostic and Statistical Manual of Mental Disorders*, 5th edition, published by the American Psychiatric Association in 2013, is a reference work classifying all the mental health conditions.
3 The extended version of Ella's story was published in our book *Life to Be Lived* (Proot & Yorke, 2014, pp. 29–30).

References

Clark, D., 2014. 'Total Pain': The Work of Cicely Saunders and the Maturing of a Concept. [Online] Available at: http://endoflifestudies.academicblogs.co.uk/total-pain-the-work-of-cicely-saunders-and-the-maturing-of-a-concept [Accessed 4 May 2020].

Frankl, V., 2004. Man's Search for Meaning: The Classic Tribute to Hope from the Holocaust. London: Rider.

Hartley, N. et al., 2010. Creativity in Palliative Care. London: St Christopher's Hospice.

How to Die: Simon's Choice, 2016. [Film] Directed by R. Deacon. United Kingdom: BBC.

Mayne, M., 2006. The Enduring Melody. London: Darton, Longman & Todd.

Proot, C. & Yorke, M., 2014. Life to Be Lived: Challenges and Choices for Patients and Carers in Life-threatening Illnesses. Oxford: Oxford University Press.

Prouty, G., 1994. Theoretical Evolutions in Person-Centred/Experiential Therapy: Applications to Schizophrenic and Retarded Psychoses. New York: Praeger.

Sabbage, S., 2016. The Cancer Whisperer: How to Let Cancer Heal Your Life. London: Coronet.

Saunders, C., 2003. Watch With Me: Inspiration for a Life in Hospice Care. Sheffield: Mortal Press.

Van Werde, D. & Morton, I., 1999. The Relevance of Prouty's Pre-therapy to Dementia Care. In: I. Morton, ed., Person-Centred Approaches to Dementia Care. Bicester: Winslow Press.

Part II

Medicine and care at the end of life

Chapter 3

Medical intervention, a life saver or a life changer?

When talking about medical intervention we think of the life-support machine, artificial feeding or other methods that prolong life. When is a life support machine to be switched off? What criteria can be put forward and with what certainty or consensus? Indeed, if criteria include that the patient is brain dead, medical opinions differ about the assessment of a patient's personal awareness and experience when they are in coma and about their capacity when recovering to respond to what life can offer, even if it is more restricted than what it was. This produces a moral issue over transferring responsibility over life and death and is in danger of becoming a negative situation, as with the 'Bland case'.[1] On the other hand, witnesses who were apparently brain dead have unexpectedly recovered and written about what they sensed when doctors thought they did not perceive anything (Moody, 1975, 2001; Giacino & White, 2005; McCullagh, 2004). These are exceptions, but they are there and encourage us to be very cautious about these matters.

Medical intervention can also take the form of regular maintenance medication or implants, and we probably all know at least one person who would not be alive if it was not for such support. Chemotherapy is the use of powerful drugs to kill off cancers, but they can and do also cause negative reactions in patients. What are the factors associated with the continuance or cessation of such treatments? Is good health a divine right to which all other life issues are seconded? Side effects, demands on patient and family, withdrawal, consequences and cost and the like need to be the subject of careful discussion and skilled management.

Sometimes in modern medicine the Hippocratic oath is being interpreted as the command to extend life regardless of the quality of that life to be lived. There is a contrast between curative medicine, in which the body is viewed as an engine which needs mending, and the care to enhance the life of the engine, seeing that it is a treasure. Medical intervention, whether by surgery or pharmacology, direct care or talking treatments make for a change in a patient's life or their view of it. It may be great or small, physical or psychological, long-lasting or brief, towards dying or recovery to some degree. Such are the questions we will consider in this chapter and the beliefs and emotions that come with them.

Quality of life and death, the purpose of medicine

Not taking anything away from the goal to save lives and heal, we feel that the aim of good medicine comes when the focus is on developing for the patient a quality of life which they can appreciate and aspire to. In doing so, especially towards the end of life, the doctor needs to remember that the family and relatives are his patients too. They need empathy for their situation and some guidance as to how to deal with the demands of anxiety and grief. A close relationship can thus be established during care which does not need to break off at the death of the patient but will probably fade out in time due to new demands of their profession and other mutual diversions of living and working.

What do we mean by quality of life?

In one sense, 'quality of life' is a neutral expression because the word 'quality' can mean good and bad. Thus, we may say 'the quality is superb' of food in a restaurant or 'the quality is much below what one comes to expect'. In medical description and particularly in palliative care, it is more specific. Health-related quality of life (HRQOL) encompasses a range of measurable aspects about health, disease, illness and medical interventions (Kaasa & Loge, 2015).

We could say that 'quality of life' stands for a full life as far as the person is able to live it – a life which enhances experience and brings hope and pleasure and a personal sense of value. This does not mean that there are never bleak or difficult periods. On the contrary, we have come across many a patient who told us that in the trial and ordeals of the illness they have found resources and experiences they did not know they had and which have helped them find new strength and meaning in their life. The following story of Maria, given to us by a palliative care physician, may help us to appreciate what 'quality of life' can be about.

> Maria, a woman with metastasised breast cancer, was celebrating an anniversary with her family. In the evening, after having enjoyed a very nice day, Maria was driven home, where she lived alone. She thought, 'If I take a box of sedatives now, there is a chance that I do not wake up in the morning. Everybody will have the memory of that nice day, and I will avoid suffering'.
>
> The next morning, neither the windows nor the doors of Maria's flat were open. The neighbours rang her daughter, wondering what was happening, because normally by this time of day her windows were open. Maria's

daughter came and found her mum in bed. She could not be woken up. She was immediately transferred to the emergency department, and it was clear that she had taken excess medication. After a couple of hours, she did wake up and confirmed that it was an unsuccessful suicide attempt, and so it was impossible to discharge Maria home, because she might make another attempt.

After consideration, we advised that Maria could stay in hospital, where care could be offered. Alternatively, she could go to a nursing home or to the palliative care unit, where specialist care was available. After 48 hours, Maria decided to go to the palliative care unit, because her cancer had metastasised and her life expectancy was only a couple of months. She also wanted to avoid unnecessary suffering.

After a week in our palliative care unit, I asked Maria whether, with hindsight, she felt she made the right decision. She confirmed she did and explained that when she was at home she had prayed every day not to wake up in the morning, but now she thanked the Lord every evening for being here and having had another good day.

Maria was amazed that her children were taking the time to come and visit her now. When she was at home, they prioritised their work, assuming that she would go on living for a long time. Now that she was 'palliative', they realised her time was limited, so they visited, sometimes with the grandchildren, who did their homework in Maria's room. They drank coffee or tea and ate cake every day. Maria was so satisfied.

This elderly lady lived for two months in the palliative care unit and developed a very close relationship with her children and grandchildren. She became very happy. Once again, as stated in the title of our first book (Proot & Yorke, 2014), there was *Life to Be Lived*. Maria had become connected again with her family, whereas before, the family members were not aware of how lonely she felt.

From Maria's and others' stories, and from personal experiences and ideas shared with us, which overlap many features mentioned in the resilience literature (Monroe & Oliviere, 2007; Hildon et al., 2010), we consider that the following aspects could be present in a person enjoying good quality of life:

1   The capacity to relate to others with the energy required to do so
2   The capacity to have realistic ambitions with the will and effort to achieve them, thus bringing a sense of achievement, however modest
3   The capacity to recognise positive and negative possibilities and to have the will to make a judgement in relation to them about personal responses and priorities
4   The awareness of other people's values and feelings as well as being able to develop one's own for the good

5   The capacity to appreciate and contribute, however modestly, to the world around, including the recognition of the messages of beauty, nature and the arts

6   Health standards appropriate to one's age and condition and balanced with a general energy and ability to adjust to and accept them – e.g. sight and hearing are important for some, less for others

7   The control – if not absence – of pain and symptoms and confidence in those who look after them

8   Happiness, hopefulness, acceptance by others, conviviality and contentment

9   The low influence of negative stress because of familial, professional or financial reasons. One feels and is supported by others.

10 The recognition of personal identity, gifts and limitations with a sense that one has made an appropriate contribution to a community life and/or a sense of thankfulness for one's own life and those who have supported it in a range of ways

It needs mentioning that the experience of quality of life is a very subjective and personal one. As we have seen in Beatrix's story, one does not have to be 100% fit or well and successful to experience a good quality of life. The range of experience is a wide continuum, and some people at the lower end of it might be frowned upon or considered with compassion by others because they have to put up with so much pain, suffering or limitations; yet in their own experience they have a good quality of life because their life has meaning to them. Perhaps they feel on top of things, or for so many other personal reasons. Similarly, a person who by the criteria of this world is 200% successful, fit and healthy, may experience a bad quality of life and surprise the people around them by committing suicide. There are no objective certainties when we try to assess how others feel.

How do we assess quality of life in another person?

The short answer to that question is that we cannot do so with any certainty. But with informed observation and attendance, we can make a reasonable guess. A range of tools (e.g. WHOQOL, SPICT, Palliative Care Outcome Scale) have been developed to help with the assessment, and a number of publications discussing the use and validity of these tools underline how significant quality of life is in health care (Albers et al., 2010; Bausewein et al., 2011; Kaasa & Loge, 2015).

The best information about their quality of life comes from the person themselves, revealed by what they say and what they don't say, and by the coherence between the information given and the manner in which it is revealed. Attentive listening is therefore vital. Thus, we will try and note the mood and the pace of the discussion as well as what is being said. Experience and gut feelings are helpful, but they are not conclusive, as there may well be some bias arising from the questioner's position.

Quality of life is a subjective response to personal circumstances which may be rooted in the subconscious as well as in conscious experience. A person's sense of value will often be conditioned by how they have been parented, by their beliefs, by how much they were part of the community and their role and function within it, and by how their professional work as well as voluntary commitments were respected and valued by others. Such responses and feelings can therefore influence the person, especially when they are not aware of them and in particular when they are near death.

Quality of life is not only individual. Its assessment might involve the impact on and a contribution shared with the group of people in which the subject operates. Thus, someone who is depressed or feeling a failure may be misjudging how they come across to those around them. How a person copes with their depression or sense of failure may inspire others by their courage and determination. This, perhaps more often, can be seen in major illness: a bedbound patient, by the demonstration of patience or thanks towards those who help them, shares a deep warmth which they may not feel themselves. It also happens that patients find strength and purpose in this new phase of their life, as a woman of 27 with a young child said:

> Being told I have cancer has turned out to be a blessing, because it has helped me to look at my life in a much more positive and incisive way.

From quality of life to quality of death

If 'quality of life' stands for a full life as far as the person is able to live it, 'quality of death' is about accepting that death is near, being comfortable with symptoms under control, and allowing the natural death to unfold as much as possible. Here again, good communication is essential to help people understand what is happening and what may or may not be helpful. Often, for instance, people find food very important to keep death at bay, and when the patient cannot eat, they want them to be given artificial food or feel very upset when the patient is not hydrated. They do not realise that this can hinder the natural dying process and cause discomfort. Indeed, the patient may not be able to swallow, or too much fluid can cause them to become bloated while the kidneys and the heart are failing. Thus, patients can have respiratory distress because of water entering the lungs.

In the palliative care unit, when food and fluid are restricted, lung oedema and swollen legs with fluid seeping out do not occur. Similarly, some treatments are better stopped towards the end of life. A palliative care physician shared:

> It is important that physicians learn to manage multi-organ failure, to recognise it and not try to correct it, because it cannot be corrected. Doctors sometimes have to decide to stop an intervention, a certain medication for instance, because the correction is causing more burden to the patient than relief. With greater technical capacity, physicians need to be critical and know the limitations of their treatments.

Complementary to medicine's art of curing and treating, nursing practices demonstrate the art of caring. The holistic focus and the time and space offered to patient and family are at the heart of this difference, as the following story of a Hospice at Home nurse illustrates.

> Leo was referred to Hospice at Home very late in his illness. When we rang the doorbell and the door opened, we could feel the frost in the air. Angela, Leo's wife, looked as though she was thinking, 'Oh Lord, more of these health professionals. I have just seen one lot out. I don't need this'. However, very reluctant body language to the fore, Angela let us in, trying to keep us in the hall and preventing us going any further.
>
> With sensitive and respectful communication about who we were, we asked if there was anything we could do to help. At first the response was negative, and then I said, absolutely checking out Angela's permission, that it was Friday afternoon, and would she want us to have a quick look to see how things were, and whether there was anything we could do so that she could manage things over the week-end. She let us in. We sat at the end of the bed and Angela next to her husband. I was quite shocked because I did not expect Leo to be on the brink of death, and this poor woman was a bit like a guard dog, trying to keep everyone out.
>
> We were very careful. This was about this couple and their wishes, and Angela very much made it plain that this was their moment, their intimate time for Leo and her. She was as tight as tight could be. We asked a few gentle questions and inquired about whether the couple were on their own over the week-end and whether they had any family. When asked whether she had ever been through anything like this before, Angela denied. I offered to talk about what might happen so that she would know what to do if things became difficult over the week-end.
>
> Through quiet observations about the catheter and other things we noticed, we were let in. Leo had not moved for 48 hours, so we explained that when patients do not move, the heels or the sacrum can get very uncomfortable, and wondered whether it might be helpful if we moved him. Gradually, we built up trust, and Angela ended up disclosing quite a lot of their story

and about Leo as a person. With her permission we did some catheter care, moved Leo and talked about how the mouth can be uncomfortable. There was an extraordinary picture of Angela straddled over her husband with arms and legs, kissing him tenderly whilst we were doing the care.

In a snapshot visit, although two or three hours long, Angela moved from a position of not wanting the nurses in the front door to being completely open to their help and support. The visit centred on Angela. It was about what was going to help and acknowledging that this was their very special time, and Leo and Angela needed to see this through, with a discreet help of the nurses where needed. When the nurses left, Angela thanked them for coming, saying how much she had learned.

Despite a difficult beginning, the nurses have facilitated Angela's understanding and acceptance of the process of dying. She felt in a better position to manage what was to come next. She knew what the changes might be and what to do with these changes up to the death. It was all right. Leo died the next day. What a blessing that they had fitted in that visit on Friday and that it went the way it did!

Everything about palliation and end of life is very complex. There is not one solution that fits all – that is not possible. Such is the trade-mark for quality of death and good terminal care. It is a never-ending challenge to look for what is important for this individual patient at this moment in time, and people are changing their minds continuously. What we think now will be different from what we thought five years ago. And the patients can change their minds too. We are in a continuously changing environment, so strategies need to be adapted continuously to what is happening in the community and what is morally acceptable for today.

Professional identity and evidence-based practice

Forever an art, in recent decades medicine has developed into a complex science. Criteria and protocols for treatment guide what doctors may or can do. A series of 'Standards, Options and Recommendations', as they are known in the medical world, are continuously being developed and updated. Based on research and clinical studies, they support the physician's thinking and decision making in the complexity of possible clinical situations and the multiplicity of available therapeutic options.

A change in appreciation of their personal and professional authority can threaten the relationship between the doctor, his role and the patient. Trained to answer questions and exercise control, some doctors are uncomfortable with an erosion of the traditional boundaries that protected them. However, personal warmth and contact between patient and doctor do not necessarily undermine scientific expertise; on the contrary, they bring it into perspective and can enhance it.

Illnesses and ill people

Fifty years ago, the physician relied on his knowledge-based diagnostic intuition to decide on the best treatment option, adapting it by trial and error. Nowadays, scientific research, statistics and technology articulate an evidence-based practice: 'In the light of these parameters, you apply this treatment'. Although helpful sometimes in clarifying what may be happening, codified diagnoses and evidence-based practice do not always account for the whole picture of a specific patient and their illness. A physician shared:

> Evidence-based practice is based on similarity, with the assumption that everyone is fairly similar. So if a patient is helped by a medicine for pain or breathlessness, it is assumed that other patients will respond to the medication in reasonably the same way. While this is often the case, it is not always so. Some patients can tolerate high doses of morphine, whereas others find even low doses cause them unacceptable side effects. It is fair to say also that a lot of medicine is still not evidence based. Experience from the wisdom of past doctors, agreed best current practice and the doctor's individual distilled experience can still play a part.

This is particularly true in psychological and spiritual distress, in which individuality and difference, which are not neatly codifiable, play an even more important part. Overdiagnosis can lead to an unfounded certainty which affects how people are being treated and considered. One diagnosis in the DSM-5,[2] for example, is 'social anxiety disorder'. It describes a pattern of behaviour which tells us that a person feels anxious in social circumstances and tries to avoid them. Is this diagnosis precise enough to understand what a patient is experiencing and how to help them? There might be any number of reasons for such behaviour which could be explored. We can hardly consider that 'social anxiety' has the same diagnostic solidity as 'appendicitis' or 'myocardial infarction', but it burdens a person with a medical label.

Another example in the realm of palliative care is 'terminal restlessness syndrome', which is often treated by heavy sedation. All it actually means is that a person is close to death and is restless; hardly a diagnosis! A palliative care physician commented how he has seen many such restless patients dramatically relieved by placing a urinary catheter. . . . They were in urinary retention and, being semi-conscious, couldn't tell the nurses. It proves to say that it is always worth searching for what might be the reason for or the meaning of a patient's restlessness.

Standards, options, recommendations . . . and much more

Physicians are educated to make a diagnosis and to follow it up by an action: if you have hypertension, then you give a drug; if there is cardiac arrest, you have to reanimate; if the patient has low haemoglobin, then you give a transfusion; if there is pneumonia, then you give antibiotics, etc. That is true in acute medicine, but in the twilight of life, patients are all chronic, with multi morbidity, and doctors need to have conversations with the patient to enquire about what their wishes and priorities are now.

A palliative care consultant of a university hospital has the strong belief that one is a product of their history so he encourages medical students to look at this particular family, to look beyond this treatment they can offer and to consider what is behind that treatment. He has the following story:

> Last Wednesday Jenny, a lady of 84 came to me, yellow, sent by the GP. The CT scan showed bile duct cancer[3] without liver metastases and without nodes. Jenny had never been sick before. She was working in agriculture. She was alone, no husband, no children, and she was still keeping cows, aged 84. At this advanced age Jenny still took her car for a MOT, and now she had come to me with bile duct cancer.
>
> I told Jenny that I thought her cancer could be operable. I asked her what she thought about that option, saying that it would mean a pancreatectomy including a part of the small guts, reanastomosis (surgery by which after part of the gut has been removed, the divided gut is reunited), hospitalisation for a couple of weeks and a risk of complications. I also told Jenny that if she decided against having the operation, there was a chance that she may not survive the next three months or even less. However, at 84 and living alone, Jenny had to think about it. I promised I would contact the surgeon to ask him to look at the images and to meet her if she would like that. He would inform Jenny about the surgical possibilities and also the burden of treatment.
>
> When I spoke to the surgeon on the phone, he immediately said that we would have to drain the bile. I replied that the first thing we had to do was to decide whether there was a possibility to do an operation and that, to this end, he would need to see the patient and look at the images. Only then could he decide to do a gallbladder drainage. If, on the other hand, it was decided that there should be no operation, then we would not have to do anything. Thus, the patient would go in liver failure, and she would be sleeping; she would go in her sleep, and that is a good death. If we drained the bile, we may prolong Jenny's life only for more suffering. The surgeon was surprised, as he admitted he did not think like that. I told him that Jenny would be coming that afternoon to see him so that he could check whether she was fit enough to have that surgery, and only after that decision would we decide about having the drainage done or not.

A true follower of the Standards-Options-Recommendations model, the surgeon said that they would have to drain the bile. The palliative care consultant surprised him, seeing the bigger picture. Doctors do not have the capacity to predict exactly what will happen to an individual patient. They can only base their predictions on statistics, and a statistical appreciation is not possible for the individual. That is the problem. But they can and should explain to the patient that they are only human beings and that they have some possibilities in treatment and maybe also some limitations. The palliative care consultant continues:

> Jenny said that she respected that I had so honestly said that surgery was an option but that to do nothing and have just a good death was another. She reflected honestly that 84 is a good age, and she had been so lucky not to suffer for her whole life, and everything had been good. So what about that next year? It could be difficult.
>
> Jenny had just one sister, a widow of five years, who was living alone now, and they were very close. She then asked whether they had to decide as sisters together or not and asked me what I would advise. I replied that I would go to the surgeon and listen to what his possibilities are, for instance whether it is an easy or a very difficult operation, and then I would go home and reflect on it and decide, looking into my heart, at what my gut feeling was.

It was clear that the physician could not decide for Jenny, but he had done his duty to inform her of the issues as well as he could.

Summarising her view on evidence-based practice and quality of life in the way she practices, a young GP considers that trying to find out what the patient's reality and aspirations are is still very much the doctor's responsibility. Beyond that, what treatment or medication is available is very much regulated and codified, but the doctor needs to exercise his judgement also. For good-quality practice, the doctor has to integrate the evidence and the guidelines as well as the reality of the patient and make a good mix of them. In doing so, the most important thing for doctors is to communicate about what they are doing, even the medical decisions, and particularly when they make mistakes. She had the following story:

> Nicole had very severe stomach pain. I gave her medication for the stomach because I thought it was a stomach inflammation. Two days later it appeared to be cholecystitis, an inflammation of the gallbladder. I knew the clinical image was not that clear when I saw her the first time; it was much clearer two days later. This is when I felt I needed to call Nicole to talk about this. I told her I felt a bit worried about her and wondered whether I had missed something. Yet I didn't think I did because it wasn't that clear when I first saw her. I needed to tell her that and check what she thought and felt.

That sort of communication is very important, particularly in palliative care. Most complaints about doctors are related to issues of communication, not clinical competency (Fong Ha & Longnecker, 2010). Physicians are not machines; they are just doctors making judgements on clinical decision guidelines. The government cannot expect them to be just robots following rules and algorithms, nor can anybody else for that matter. That is not how they work. Good communication is important at every step on the journey, from diagnosis to end, and will help decide on the best course of action to treat not merely illnesses but ill people.

Weighing up the benefits and harm of a treatment

Amongst our informants, experiences of weighing up the benefits and the harm of a treatment are mixed. A nurse has worked with physicians who carefully examined each individual situation. At the other end of the spectrum, a GP felt she was left to pick up the pieces when an oncologist suggested another line of chemotherapy which might add a number of months to the patient's life, but most of them would need to be spent in hospital, and with pain or discomfort.

In acute situations in the intensive care unit, for example, treatment may be stopped because physiologically, doctors know that the treatment they have tried does not work and the patient is dying. When this happens, in many ICUs, care is taken to remove everything that is not serving the comfort of the patient and is not useful in the dying process. That is quite normal and sensible. If, for some reason, such as keeping beds filled, doctors were to continue a treatment they know is failing, this would be crossing a serious ethical boundary. Out of respect for the dying person, we also have to let the person die. For other illnesses, in oncology for example, whether treatment works or not depends on many factors. If, after a while, they see that a treatment does not work, oncologists will try something else; they progress step by step. Sometimes wrong decisions are made. A GP recalls:

> A patient was artificially fed after severe brain damage. There was no contact anymore with the patient, and without any good discussion with the family or thoughts about the options, they put in the feeding line. The patient lasted for more than a year, simply staring. There was no eye contact, nothing. For the family it was horrible.
>
> This is an example of an accident of medicine; it is not good medicine. In some conditions, it can be good to feed somebody artificially, but only for a period of time and when recovery is possible. In other conditions, doctors have to be compassionate and not force people to live in an artificial way.
>
> These are always very difficult decisions, and we should not make them on our own. They should be taken in a team so the pros and cons can be discussed and a balanced way of being with the decision is achieved when the time comes to talk to the family.

Sometimes the oncologist sees the glass half empty while the surgeon sees it half full, and the patient is all too keen to go along with the latter and believe it is half full. The patient is going to die anyway, but the surgeon is willing to try something, and he can affirm that since he has started practising this intervention, he has managed on average to prolong the life of his patients by three months. However, there is no information on the quality of life of those patients nor how they understood this. Did they believe they were going to live for three months or five years, or did they think they were cured?

Codified practice tends to shift the focus from the ill person to the illness and change the doctor–patient relationship. A UK GP commented:

> I think quite a bit has shifted over the 40 years of my qualifying. Nowadays, I wonder if people who have incurable disease are offered treatment which will not cure them, whether it gives them a false sense of optimism as to where they realistically are. I think that has clouded the whole issue of what is fair and honest quite badly. In the old days, I could go and see Mrs X who was dying, and have a really blunt conversation asking whether she would want me to get the vicar to come in. She'd reply asking how long I thought she had left, and when I said that it could be this week, she'd plan to have Communion the next day, asking whether I could get the hairdresser to come in first.

It happens much less often now that a doctor has a conversation along these lines with a dying patient. More often, conversations are about treatment options and possibilities. But even so, much depends on how doctors communicate with their patients. A palliative care specialist and radio-oncologist feels he is the only one who says clearly to the patient that there are two paths: 'more treatment' and 'end of life'.

> Oscar came in for antalgic (i.e. pain-reducing) irradiation[4] and then said he was due to start another course of chemotherapy the next week. Surprised, I reminded Oscar that he had already had three schemes of chemotherapy in the last twelve months, and they had all failed . . . But, he said, they will be trying a new drug. I asked whether he realised that a tumour that had not reacted to the previous three schemes might not react to the fourth one either. He was aware of that, but he was going for a cure.
>
> I pressed Oscar, asking whether he really thought that was possible and whether he had asked his oncologist what the chances were that this Phase One trial[5] might work. I pursued to tell him that in general, in a Phase One study, there is less than 5% treatment effectiveness and that the research is mostly looking for toxicity, and I asked him whether he realised that.

I then had to say that if he needed it for psychological reasons, he could go for that treatment, but in the meantime, he had to consider the 95% chance that it would not be effective. So he needed to look at what was important for him in order to fulfil end-of-life issues such as: did he need to say goodbye to somebody, did he have to forgive somebody, did he have to organise something for his children, for his partner, elderly parents?

You have to look at both paths: on the one hand, what is needed if the treatment is not effective, and on the other hand, start the treatment if you need it for psychological reasons and hope that you are in the 5% for whom the treatment is effective.

Medicine is trying to push back the boundaries of what it can do, and exactly because of that, it becomes more and more important for physicians to be aware of what medicine cannot do and to stop treatment in time. Is it good to artificially feed patients with dementia into eternity? What is the point of keeping all the coma patients in coma rooms? A palliative care consultant said:

We discussed with our palliative care team how we manage the problem of the patients who have chronic diseases with all the side effects of treatments that are more and more important. These patients are suffering increasingly, and eventually a time comes where they say they cannot live this life any longer. That is when the physician is utterly disappointed, because they have done so much for this patient.

For instance, after a bone marrow transplant a patient may develop a graft-versus-host reaction, whereby the graft is not accepted and the body is making antibodies against the graft. The patient then develops skin problems, rash, mucosal problems, and their appetite decreases. The patient is unwell and suffering, and the efforts to solve the problem remain without any result. Finally, after one or two years, the patient is disappointed, because the promise to be cured with the bone marrow transplant is not fulfilled. So they cannot stand the suffering any longer and are contemplating euthanasia.

For the haematologist this is not acceptable. From their perspective, there is no tumour, so in effect the patient is cured. Thus, we end up with patients who are living with a lot of disadvantages and side effects, missing out on quality of life and no longer feeling able to live that life. But the physician does not hear the question, and within the palliative care team, we wonder how we can support these patients, who come to us more and more frequently.

Situations like this happen not only to bone marrow transplant patients but also to patients with heart failure and COPD (chronic obstructive pulmonary disease). People with renal failure are visiting the hospital three times a week for dialysis, which means that three days in the week, they do not feel good! They are spending a lot of time at the hospital, and they are not well. When do we decide to stop the dialysis? What can be the process of making the decision to stop? The nephrologists will say, "As long as we continue, the patient will live". But who is listening to what is the quality of life for that patient? We have been told of a person who was in this situation, and the only way he could escape the doctor's urging to keep going in to dialysis was to fail to keep his appointments, and so he died. It can be very comfortable for physicians to start another treatment. They give the patient hope, and they do not have to discuss all the issues about end of life.

When a treatment is possible, can be paid for etc., one can still question its appropriateness, wondering whether the consequences make it right and whether patients are in a position to decide for or against having the treatment. A GP said how she can often be entangled in such questions when the specialist in the hospital suggests chemotherapy after chemotherapy.

> Patients come to talk to us about this suggestion for another chemotherapy. I know it will not make any difference, the patient will be sick and tired, but who am I to say that? That is very difficult. Sometimes I dare ask a patient whether they really want this treatment and why. I try to explore where they are. Sometimes a patient will say that actually he does not want it anymore, but his wife does, and this opens a whole new line of communication. It is not our responsibility to decide, but I think it is our responsibility to help the patient see more clearly why they are making the decision they are making.

It is essential, in our view, and more generally good practice that decisions about prolonging life or ending it by medical intervention are related to a clear ethical and practical stance which is shared within the multiprofessional team and communicated to the patient and their family. A university physician notes:

> I have been a member of the ethical committee of the hospital for 20 years. Our stance is that if a patient on the stroke unit has a haemorrhage or an embolic phenomenon in the brain, and the patient is not conscious, we start immediate treatment, and we do everything that makes recovery possible. But in advance we say that if there is no sign of recovery after three months, we will stop the treatment.
> We will do everything we can to help the patient and the family, but if after three months nothing is changing for the patient, we will stop the treatment. We are not committing ourselves to situations like Premier Sharon in Israel,

who was kept 'alive' for three years. That is not life. If there is no chance that there is some degree of consciousness, then further treatment is useless. So we avoid that, and we are clear with the family about the goal of treatment and the procedures.

However, we do state this policy from the very beginning. We have to inform the family and communicate with them, saying this is the basis of the agreement, and every week we will discuss the progress and see how it flows, keeping an eye on the goal.

We are touched by the sense of comfort we get thinking that as a family of a coma patient, we might be treated in such a way with regular support and meeting with the team but also advance warning that there may be a cutting-off point and what the criteria for that cutting-off point are.

A technical and an ethical act

There is a moral issue in intervening in a person's life, especially if it leads to continuance of life or its end. Is it right to maintain or revive a life at all costs? If not, where are the limits, and are they unique to human beings? If so, why? Is it because of spirituality, of soul, a deep psychological bond, usefulness to the world, however limited? What about a beloved dog or horse? Both are highly intelligent creatures, and many would say they fulfil the above questions. One informant told us:

We just lost a very dear and much-loved dog and went through a beauti-ful process with her. The vet had warned the time would come when we would have to put her down. The extraordinary thing was that we did not wrestle with any moral issues at all. Her dying was handled beautifully, and it was highly emotional, particularly for my wife. I remember thinking in ret-rospect about what the difference is between the dog and a friend. Why can we make the decision so easily for an animal, in moral terms? Perhaps the answer is because the dog cannot talk to us, so we do not know what his views are, and the dog is not a human. But then why do we have to make that distinction?

What is unique about being a person, which is not the same question as to whether that person is unique? Is human uniqueness based on the capacity to express oneself? To produce and contribute to society? To be a consumer? To be in relationship? To make choices? Somehow, the vast majority of people seem to have a deep sense about human uniqueness, but they cannot define what they really mean by it, let alone agree on that meaning. The ethical call to do well for the patient cannot be avoided. But what is well? Is there a liability for specific malpractice or incompetent prescribing?

What makes medical intervention right or wrong?

If medical intervention is an ethical act as well as a technical one, what then makes it right or wrong? Does the informed decision of a patient to want to draw their life to a close, together with somebody else taking the responsibility to share that decision, make it right? And if so, who is to decide? What might be the form of a third-party role, what knowledge and criteria should they have to apply?

Some people feel overwhelmingly that if the experience of loving support and closeness with putting down a dog can be replicated in the case of a human relationship, with the proper criteria and real emotional support, that that must be right; that must be permissible. And in some countries, there are legal provisions to allow euthanasia under certain conditions. What is the difference between the dog's death, the death of a child who is grievously ill in the womb or that of a child who is unwanted by a fornicating parent? What is the difference? Why can some people nod in the case of abortion pretty well on demand and agonise over assisted dying in an aged adult? Such reflection can be very unsettling. The human mind seeks to set priorities, and the main issue can become lost in the thinking, the discussion and the aims.

A key criterion could be our valuation of the person or creature concerned, whether by compassion or for its intrinsic value. Medical intervention in the treatment of a very valuable horse, for instance, will be much more likely than for a hack, a horse perceived of little financial or emotional value. Still, just because we approach such valuation in different ways, the human's ability to communicate and the fact that the people around the patient may feel a need to come to a judgement about whether the patient wishes to die or not is very thorny. How can people do that? The patient's wishes may be expressed, but when the situation arises, they may have changed their mind. Or their wishes are not expressed, and one finds oneself in a position of great responsibility in making any assumptions about it. Even when one considers the power of love as a cause for action, that can be very sensitive, but it can also be very cruel to be kind. People may have to live with the decisions they made at such a critical time for a very long time afterwards. Quite a thorn!

In a secularised world where self-determination is the highest value, it is absolutely necessary and it is the biggest dream of every secularised person to be in control of their life. For some that means that in an ideal world we should have, like we have a vending machine for Coca-Cola and so on, we should have machines where you can have your suicide pill. You want it, you push it, you have it. It's your decision. And reality is not far away from that 'ideal', as you can order certain drugs from China or Mexico on line.

This can be the consequence of a secularised society. If there is no room for transcendence – whatever you call that transcendence – then the only thing that people have is themselves. They are at the steering wheel and have to have the right to do what they like. And actually, at this point in time, a lot of people may see the fact that they have to ask a physician, 'Please terminate my life', as paternalistic. Why should the physician have to agree? They feel that people should be able to decide and do it themselves.

But then come the problems: if people over 70 have this kind of pill, who will make sure that the pill is not taken by mistake by the grandchild or given to somebody else? There is no capacity to control, and we come to a situation of which Daniel Callahan suggests not to allow something that you cannot control (Callahan, 2012). For him, the main issue is that there will be abuses, so we need to protect people, and the best way to protect them is to make sure that 'officially' it is not possible to happen. We all have red lights. That means that we have to stop. But sometimes we have to drive through it. If we see a lorry coming down the hill and we see it is not going to stop, we have to drive through the red light. Nevertheless, it is not because some people sometimes drive through them that we should abolish the red lights.

We are left with more questions than answers when we consider the increasing trend in our post-modern society for killing to become accepted or even to be considered a medical act. Who guarantees the responsibility of society to provide care for their older, dying and vulnerable citizens when euthanasia and physician-assisted dying become the norm? Could a local ethical and support group provide protection for the elderly and infirm? Would a 'ward-of-court system' be strong enough? And what about the risk of conflict between personal and professional values of physicians and other health care professionals and the legal requirements they are expected to enforce?

Accountability, liability and risk

In an environment of uncertainty, compromise and consensus, the shift in focus of the medical profession from personal professional judgement to codified practices has far-reaching consequences. An older physician shared:

> Medicine is no longer an art with its trial and error. Everything in this country is evidence-based. So if the evidence says the doctor should do this and you don't do it, you will be sued. If you do this and the evidence says it does not work, somebody will make a complaint. Once in defensive gear, everybody is like rabbits in the headlights of a car. So I could be your doctor, and you could say you had enough of this and cannot go on, and I would have to say there is nothing I can do to help. If you refused treatment, you would be asked to sign a piece of paper. It is about liability, and that clouds the whole issue of medical intervention.

Codified practice can exercise complete control over the way doctors think, and their responsibility as professionals can be greatly reduced. A trend which is enhanced by increasing complexity and liability. Most senior doctors are strongly insured against this liability, because many patients are willing to pursue issues relating to failures in surgery and treatments, even when there is no evidence of incompetence or lack of care. Differing opinions in a family feed this liability culture, which has a negative impact on risk taking. The following story illustrates this:

> Harry was sitting on the beach with the family, and the tide had gone out, and suddenly there was a person running up the beach, saying a girl was being swept out to sea. The sea was very rough, but as they were the only people with a boat, Harry went out. Within two minutes the boat was damaged in the waves but he found the girl and pulled her up into his boat. He thought they were not going to make it. Harry's wife, sitting on the beach, thought along these lines too and she took the children away from the beach so they would not watch Daddy drowning. Anyway, Harry made it back to the beach and walked home, and the family of the girl he saved agreed to pay to have his boat mended. When he sent them the bill as arranged, he received a letter from a lawyer saying that if he pursued that family anymore, he would be sued for harassment!

The important thing transposing Harry's situation to the end of life is that a patient can say to a doctor, 'I really want you to end my life' and so he does, but the patient's sister, brother, husband, wife or son can turn around and say that the patient would never have allowed that. Doing what one considers to be the 'right' thing can cause resentment with others, and the doctor could be called to court and go to prison. We are left wondering whether this liability culture is an expression of society's and people's denial of the inevitability of death and mortality, aptly reinforced by modern ways of trying to make money out of people's dreams and fears.

Alongside legislation about patients' rights, there is a wide-spread movement towards advance care planning to support the patient's choice and autonomy and clarify the doctor's responsibility. People are encouraged to make a 'living will' in which to indicate what they want and what they do not want in certain situations of declining health. With a living will, medical and caring professions, as well as potential patients and relatives, have some peace of mind knowing what is going to happen. However, it remains a difficult issue, as not all forms have legal standing, people can quite reasonably change their minds or priorities over time, or the living will may not be at hand to state the wish of the patient not to be resuscitated when the paramedics are there.

Interpretations differ among physicians about how to work with a living will. Some take the patient's request and decision as a point of reference for their autonomy and are inclined to comply with their personal preference without even having to think about it. Others make it the starting point of holistic care, beginning with a comprehensive assessment and communication, trying to understand the motives and attitudes behind the patient's wish. Indeed, people can quite reasonably change their minds or priorities over time.

Another huge question which leaves scope for misunderstandings and failure is the one of accountability. Who is taking responsibility for a medical intervention? And more generally, who is in charge of the care for a patient? Who takes overall responsibility when multiple problems involve as many specialties? One of our interviewees told us the story of Conny and Lisa:

> Lisa's daughter Conny is monstrously handicapped and is bouncing in and out of hospital with repeated infections. Just over 20 years old, and Conny can't see, and she can't hear or communicate. She was recently in a huge amount of pain, and I managed to get her admitted to the local hospice for a few weeks, and they couldn't sort it. On one home visit, the GP said to Lisa, "Goodness me, I did not believe in euthanasia until I met your daughter!"
>
> Lisa felt quite relieved to hear the GP be so honest. It is so difficult and so painful. They are anticipating Conny's death all the time. She now has 24-hour care, but Lisa is quite difficult to help. She is very tense, there is a lot of anger, but she is very open, and she has talked to me about how it might be for her daughter at the end of life. They live in an area where the support is abysmal. In fact, there isn't any. The GPs won't go out at night, and no one GP takes responsibility for Conny's care. I tried to encourage the hospice to set up an advance care plan, but it hasn't worked. I have even offered to go to the meetings as a friend just to support Lisa.
>
> No one will take responsibility. Conny has a neurologist and a palliative care consultant, but no one is taking the lead in coordinating her care. The GP surgery has pretty much shut down. Conny is somewhat in a black hole out there. She has a learning-disability nurse, a community matron, but there is no one to coordinate her different care needs.
>
> I have written letters for Lisa when she has not known what to do, and then Lisa will modify them because she does not want to cause trouble. I feel helpless. I cannot force myself in on the situation even though I do think I could help resolve it.

What can they do for Conny? She is in crying pain, and no one seems able to alleviate her suffering. On top of that, Conny's needs are so complex that there is need to oversee and coordinate her care, but no one is taking responsibility. Maybe they are afraid of getting overinvolved in their efforts to help? Or they are not willing to risk liability when so much could go wrong. Or there is no regulatory framework for considering this their priority.

Matching patient's motivation and treatment

We were fortunate to meet a palliative care physician whose attitude struck us as being centred around the patient's quality of life. He told us how he always discusses treatment with the patient to see what is useful and whether this is what they are prepared to accept, giving the following example.

> Norman, an 80-year-old patient with lung cancer, asks the doctor whether he can do something so that he might celebrate his 50th wedding anniversary in four months' time. They have set a date, the venue is booked, the catering bespoke. So he asks the doctor to help him keep that celebration date clear. The doctor's answer is yes, of course. They will do everything that is possible. Even if, in his medical opinion, it is likely to enhance suffering, they will do everything they can to optimise Norman's day. Sometimes that can be achieved by giving the patient steroids to have a good appetite and to be a little euphoric so that they enjoy the occasion.
>
> Next door, another 80-year-old patient with lung cancer and a life expectancy of about three months tells the doctor that his wife died five years ago, he does not have any children, is alone, and pleads with the doctor to do nothing to prolong his life but to let him die peacefully. The sooner he could be with his wife again, the better.

Although suffering a similar diagnosis, both men are very different, and treatment can be made to match these differences as much as possible. Because there is increasing capacity to intervene medically, even with a potentially positive outcome, it does not mean that it is always necessarily right to do so in a particular situation.

Some doctors, unfortunately, did not learn how to listen to the patient and try and find out what their priorities are. They come with their agenda. A palliative care physician suggests:

> We have to give the patient responsibility and enquire about what their wishes and their priorities are now. Would they like to extend their life span? Generally, they will say no. It is not so much the length but the quality of life that matters most. But if we look at the research in medicine, we are always researching which treatment gives the longest survival time.

In this physician's opinion, the real question doctors have to consider again and again is 'What is the motivation of this patient?' He tells the story of Ann.

> Ann requested that I make a note in her file expressing her firm decision not to be given chemotherapy again. As asked, I wrote it down in her file. Six months later Ann came to see me again and told me that her daughter was three months pregnant. She asked whether I could do something for her so that she could see her first grandchild, due in six months' time. I replied that I could, but that she would need some chemotherapy to prolong her life. She wanted to start the next morning. I said we could do so, in spite of the fact that I had written in her notes, on her request, not to give her any more chemotherapy.

Even though people make a living will and make their wishes clear in advance decisions, they can change their minds. Ann now had a new priority – seeing the birth of her grandchild – so they changed the plan and started treatment. This is palliative treatment in practice, i.e. attuned to serving the patient's quality of life by matching the treatment plan to their motivation for the treatment and, more generally, for their life. The following moving story puts this in an even starker perspective:

> Seven-year-old Amy suffered from osteosarcoma, a highly malignant bone tumour, with metastases. Amy's mother Georgina, who was 30 weeks pregnant, came to ask whether we could do some radiation for Amy. She hoped that with the treatment Amy could survive four more months so that, for some weeks at least, Georgina would have two children. In the likelihood that Amy might die sooner rather than later, Georgina feared that her new child to be born would be replacing her daughter if we did not do anything.
> Keen to take Georgina's request into consideration as well as Amy's comfort, we told Georgina that we would irradiate the very dangerous localisations, not everything, so as to avoid suffering due to the treatment while trying to prolong Amy's survival. A special agreement was made for the irradiation of Amy, and Georgina drove 100 km to and from the hospital for Amy to have that treatment, because all the other units closer to home had refused.

Amy's situation shows that the whole family is the patient and that the doctor's response is not only guided by the patient. The treatment must be feasible from a medical point of view, and there needs to be some reasonable chance that the result that is asked for can be obtained. Amy's physician is not in favour of prolonging life simply to prolong it. However, if there is a higher priority for the patient or, in this case, for the mother, then he feels he has to consider it. He would not normally irradiate lung metastases, even if they were involving the thoracic wall, except to alleviate terrible pain. But, in the circumstances, a local irradiation could avoid a pleural effusion and give Amy a more comfortable and probably a longer life. So he decided he would go for it so that Georgina could possibly for a while experience having two children.

Sometimes the motivation of the patient is not straightforward, and one needs to listen to the question behind the question. A Belgian physician tells the following story:

> Irene came to see me three years ago about a recurring breast cancer which had spread all over the thoracic wall and was resistant to all hormonal and chemotherapeutic possibilities. Irene asked whether her situation placed her within the criteria of the euthanasia law. I replied that she was fulfilling all the criteria and asked what her wish was. She said, "I cannot understand that my husband still loves me. He needs another woman with whom he could live normally. That is not possible with me now".
>
> I told Irene that it occurred to me that she was looking at what was important for her husband but that I wondered what was important for herself. She replied that she had a daughter of 20 who was studying to be a nurse and was a year away from graduation. Her wish was to support her daughter for that last year and to see her employed, independent and self-supporting. Recognising that this was her wish, I asked whether we should try and go for it.
>
> Irene replied that her treating physician had told her that because of prior irradiation, there was no more possibility for further such treatment. Despite my colleagues' conviction that further treatment was useless, I told Irene that if she would like to support her daughter for another year, I was prepared to try more irradiation to help her achieve this goal.
>
> We did that very complex treatment, the tumour disappeared, and Irene survived 16 more months. Her daughter had finished her studies and was employed as a nurse by the time of Irene's death. When Irene spent the last week of her life in the hospital, she asked for me to be called to the ward, because she wanted to thank me. Aware that if she had not met me, nobody would have tried to prolong her life, she wanted me to know how precious it had been for her and her daughter to have that time together.

The lesson of Irene's story is that it was not because the patient is asking for treatment but because of their motivation for the treatment that the physician offered to go ahead with it. If the patient is motivated and has a goal, then they are committed. In those circumstances, he feels, doctors need to be committed too.

> ## To go further. . .
>
> 1   What areas would be important to you to assess and enhance quality of life and death for a patient?
> 2   *Good communication helps to treat not merely illnesses but ill people.* Do you agree or disagree? Give examples from your experience to explain why and how.
> 3   Medical intervention is a technical and an ethical act. What issues would you want to consider in evaluating the appropriateness of an intervention or treatment?

Notes

1   Anthony David "Tony" Bland (21 September 1970–3 March 1993) was a supporter of Liverpool F.C. injured in the Hillsborough disaster. He suffered severe brain damage that left him in a persistent vegetative state, as a consequence of which the hospital, with the support of his parents, applied for a court order allowing him to 'die with dignity'. As a result, he became the first patient in English legal history to be allowed to die by the courts through the withdrawal of life-prolonging treatment, including food and water.
2   *Diagnostic and Statistical Manual of Mental Disorders*, 5th edition, published by the American Psychiatric Association in 2013, is a reference work classifying all the mental health conditions.
3   Bile duct cancer, or cholangiocarcinoma, originates in the bile ducts which drain bile from the liver into the small intestine. No potentially curative treatment exists except surgery, but most people have advanced-stage disease at presentation and are inoperable at the time of diagnosis.
4   In the case of metastatic bone lesions that are painful, for instance, some irradiation can relieve the pain very effectively.
5   Phase One clinical trials are a toxicity study, looking at the doses in which a new drug is tolerable for patients and whether, in the meantime, it is effective against the tumour or not.

References

Albers, G., Echteld, M. A., de Vet, H. C. W., Onwuteaka-Philipsen, B. D., van der Linden, M. H. M. & Deliens, L., 2010. Evaluation of Quality of Life Measures for Use in Palliative Care: A Systematic Review. *Palliative Medicine*, Volume 24 (1), pp. 17–37.

Bausewein, C., Simon, S., Benalia, H., Downing, J., Mwangi-Powell, F. N., Daveson, B. A., Harding, R., Higginson, I. J. & PRISMA, 2011. Implementing Patient Reported Outcome Measures (PROMs) in Palliative Care – User's Cry for Help. *Health Quality of Life Outcomes*, Volume 9 (27). doi: 10.1186/1477-7525-9-27.

Callahan, D., 2012. *The Roots of Bioethics: Health, Progress, Technology, Death.* Oxford: Oxford University Press.

Fong Ha, J. & Longnecker, N., 2010. Doctor-Patient Communication: A Review. *The Ochsner Journal*, Volume 10 (1), pp. 38–43.

Giacino, J. & White, J., 2005. The Vegetative and Minimally Conscious States: Current Knowledge and Remaining Questions. *The Journal of Head Trauma Rehabilitation*, Volume 20, pp. 30–50.

Hildon, Z., Montgomery, S. M., Blane, D., Wiggins, R. D. & Netuveli, G., 2010. Examining Resilience of Quality of Life in the Face of Health-related and Psychosocial Adversity at Older Ages: What Is "Right" About the Way We Age? *The Gerontologist*, Volume 50 (1), pp. 36–47.

Kaasa, S. & Loge, J., 2015. Quality of Life in Palliative Care: Principles and Practice. In: N. Cherny et al., eds., *Oxford Textbook of Palliative Medicine*, 5th edition. Oxford: Oxford University Press.

McCullagh, P., 2004. *Conscious in a Vegetative State? A Critique of the PVS Concept*. Dordrecht: Kluwer Academic Publishers.

Monroe, B. & Oliviere, D., 2007. *Resilience in Palliative Care: Achievement in Adversity*. Oxford: Oxford University Press.

Moody, R. J., 1975, 2001. *Life After Life: The Investigation of a Phenomenon – Survival of Bodily Death*. New York: HarperCollins Publishers.

Proot, C. & Yorke, M., 2014. *Life to Be Lived: Challenges and Choices for Patients and Carers in Life-threatening Illnesses*. Oxford: Oxford University Press.

Chapter 4

Euthanasia and assisted dying

As medicine and the available scopes of treatment become more complex, so do the decisions in the twilight of life. Who makes those decisions is a fundamental question leading to many others. How and to what extent can or have patients to be informed, advised and consulted about treatment options and what happens to their body? Should the patient or the family have the right to demand a treatment which the doctors know to be useless or excessively expensive? Can a doctor refuse to do what they are being asked on medical and/or on personal moral grounds? If they do, how binding are their decisions, and what alternatives are there for the patient? In our consumer society, patients who have been refused a treatment can decide to go elsewhere, and different levels of treatment depending on what patients can afford are not inconceivable.

Writing against a background of increasing curiosity and specific legislation in some countries allowing life-shortening medical intervention, it felt appropriate to consider a chapter with euthanasia and assisted dying as the subject. This does not indicate an approval of these practices, but there is plenty of disagreement and constructive and strong feelings to prove how highly relevant they are to the debates about end of life in our Western society. Stories and experiences of people involved in end-of-life care both in the UK, where euthanasia and physician-assisted dying are illegal, and in the Low Countries, where it can be carried out under certain conditions, help us interpret how these attitudes and concepts affect the people of today and reflect on the impact of the law, 15 years on. We further consider how patient, family and professional make and live with end-of-life decisions, whether they result in letting nature take its course and/or in medical intervention.

Euthanasia, assisted dying, palliative sedation . . . what is it?

One of our informants asked a patient whether they were 'jumping the queue', a telling metaphor to help clarify what people mean when they talk about assisted dying. Indeed, the variety of terminology to identify interventions at the end of life adds to the general confusion, and trying to clarify what people mean seems of the utmost importance. A chaplain in a Belgian university hospital tells a striking story:

> One of the first things I have to do when people ask about euthanasia is to explain what it is and check whether that is what they want. Some elderly people will say they want euthanasia, and when I ask to clarify whether they want a doctor to come in with a syringe and kill them with that syringe, they say no. They just want to have no more pain and no more treatment, no more scans; hence, I understand that what they really want is to be left in peace. The problem with euthanasia is that when it is introduced, people understand it to be what it originally meant: 'I want a good death'. But in our country, it means a specific kind of death, and it becomes confused with all sorts of hopes and fears.

The fear of pain and suffering, the loss of autonomy and control and/or the loss of existential meaning are at the heart of people's requests in both euthanasia and palliative sedation. If it is done properly, in both processes, the doctor and/or the team prepare patient and family for what is to come, and they agree to the procedure. The main difference is one of intention which needs to be clear and unambiguous for all involved: caregivers, patient and family.

In palliative sedation substantial doses of painkillers, which may diminish the patient's consciousness, are administered, usually in the last days of life, to alleviate unbearable and unacceptable suffering for the patient in the first place and after all other means have failed to obtain the expected relief. While it may be necessary sometimes to maintain sedation until the patient's death to relieve refractory symptoms, in no way does palliative sedation seek to hasten death. A nurse has the following story:

> Charlotte needed 33 medications a day. Convinced she was a burden to her husband and children, she repeated day after day: "Let me go. I want to die. Please don't give me any more medication". She made several suicide attempts and eventually convinced the GP who referred her to the hospital for euthanasia.
>
> On the palliative care ward, combined use of painkillers and controlled sedation allowed Charlotte to rest peacefully in bed. Her adult children feared they might betray their mother's resolve for euthanasia, but we could reassure them: she was receiving no more medical treatment, and we did not do anything to prolong her life; we were only making her comfortable. Charlotte eventually died in her husband's arms, listening to the music they'd played at their wedding.

Reversible sedation can be used to prevent pain or symptoms during handling or when limiting or stopping treatment. When sedation needs to be maintained till the very end, some speak of terminal sedation. A study revealed that 7,5% of the patients ($N = 266$) admitted to a palliative care unit needed sedation at the end of life. It started on average 2,5 days before death when patients gave consent to start it because of increased suffering (Claessens et al., 2011).

In euthanasia doctor and patient have to set a time for administering a syringe that will kill the patient in a matter of minutes. Patients are on a cliff and have to decide to jump. Terminal sedation is slower, more similar to natural dying, more gradual, and its intention is to relieve the patient's pain and symptoms, not to hasten death.

Assisted dying is helping someone to die by pointing them in the direction of a website where they can find the necessary products or of an address, in Switzerland for instance, where they can be helped with assisted suicide, which is when someone prescribes or prepares a lethal cocktail which the patient has to administer himself, usually by drinking. Euthanasia and/or physician-assisted dying is when the doctor administers the lethal drug.

It is important to mention that, even in the countries where there is a specific legislation, euthanasia is not (yet?) considered a medical act just like abortion is not a medical act. This is why physicians are not obliged to carry out either of those acts. They are a criminal offence for which, provided they can prove that certain conditions have been respected, the perpetrators will not be prosecuted.

The World Medical Association[1] maintains that euthanasia and physician-assisted suicide are in conflict with basic ethical principles of medical practice and strongly encourages physicians to refrain from participating in them, even if a national law allows it or decriminalises it under certain conditions. The 38th WMA General Assembly stated:

> Euthanasia, that is the act of deliberately ending the life of a patient, even at the patient's own request or at the request of close relatives, is unethical. This does not prevent the physician from respecting the desire of a patient to allow the natural process of death to follow its course in the terminal phase of sickness.
>
> (World Medical Association, 1987)

A motion put forward by the Dutch and Canadian Medical Associations to review the 1987 resolution to a more neutral position has been withdrawn from the 2018 WMA General Assembly for lack of international support. In 2019 the 70th Assembly succeeded the 1987 statement with the following:

> The WMA reiterates its strong commitment to the principles of medical ethics and that utmost respect has to be maintained for

human life. Therefore, the WMA is firmly opposed to euthanasia and physician-assisted suicide. No physician should be forced to participate in euthanasia or assisted suicide, nor should any physician be obliged to make referral decisions to this end. Separately, the physician who respects the basic right of the patient to decline medical treatment does not act unethically in forgoing or withholding unwanted care, even if respecting such a wish results in the death of the patient.

(World Medical Association, 2019)

The WMA makes it very clear that euthanasia is an active act to kill a patient. It is to be distinguished from medical interventions at the end of life, which, performed with the intention to relieve pain and suffering and/or to respect the patient's wish, may result in the death of the patient, such as sedation, limiting, discontinuing or deescalating treatment, stopping nutrition or hydration, controlling refractory symptoms with strong opiates and emergency protocols.

Situation in the countries we considered

For clarity's sake, we would like to give a brief summary of what we have understood the situation to be in the countries we considered at the time of our interviewing. Debate is ongoing, and a number of other countries or states allow euthanasia and/or assisted dying, but we have limited our enquiry to near where we work – the United Kingdom with an excursion to Switzerland, the Netherlands and Belgium.

United Kingdom

Under no circumstances can euthanasia be practised in the UK. Palliative sedation is allowed if it can be proven that the aim of the intervention is to alleviate pain and suffering not to shorten life.

A bill on assisted dying was debated and rejected in the UK Parliament in September 2015: 118 voted for, 330 against. In 2018, on the island of Guernsey, the parliament voted against legalising assisted dying with 24 votes to 18, rather choosing to improve palliative care on the island. This was the 10th attempt to legalise euthanasia on British territory since 2003.

However, lots of questions are raised about whether to permit voluntary euthanasia with the person's consent, and the debate suffers lack of clarity and tremendous controversy. What prospect is there to achieve a secure and more common view? Who would do that? People doubt whether it is up to MPs or magistrates to decide what the public wants in terms of life expectancy, as it is such an individual prerogative. But if it were left totally to the individual, how would they go about finding a doctor who will do it?

Professionals or others may need to be on the receiving end of something that has official support and legal standing for clarity about whether and when and, eventually, how, but a lot of difficulties stand in the way of achieving it. For instance, a High Court judge in a recent case about medical intervention on a critically ill baby made the comment that he was there to interpret the law, not give his personal opinion. The result of that was that the parents wanted to appeal because they were expecting a personal view but could not get it, as the judge decided the case on the law rather than on his personal feelings.

Switzerland

Because of the lack of clarity and legal provision, some English people feel they have to go to Switzerland, where organisations exist to help foreigners with assisted suicide at a cost of about £7000.

Criteria to qualify for assisted suicide in Switzerland include suffering from an incurable illness, being sound of mind and having been thinking about it for some time. The patient's medical records are examined, and if they pass the scrutiny, a provisional green light is given.

On the eve of the intervention the patient must convince a second physician, who does an independent assessment and needs to confirm the criteria are met for the procedure to go ahead. They have to fill in forms in the place where the assisted suicide will happen. The family must be there and show understanding.

To conform to Swiss legislation the patient must administer the drug himself, and this must be filmed. Usually a lethal cocktail is prepared in an intravenous drip which a doctor or nurse will put in a vein, using a needle. The patient has to action the drip himself to start the fluids flowing into their vein.

The Netherlands

In the Netherlands euthanasia is an illegal act, but the doctor will not be prosecuted if he conforms to certain conditions. This is why all euthanasia procedures have to be reported and are reviewed by specialised committees. A number of due care criteria must be fulfilled in order to proceed with euthanasia:

1   The patient must make a voluntary request of their own free will;
2   The patient must have uncontrollable symptoms and be suffering beyond relief;
3   The physician must inform the patient about his situation and outlook;
4   There must be no possible chance of recovery;

5   An external check with a second doctor who does not know the patient and is not involved in the treatment must come to the same conclusion;
6   The procedure must be practised with due medical care.

Whenever euthanasia is considered, the process is started, which involves checking the above due care criteria, informing the forensic doctor to ask for a form, keeping a log book, having the process checked by an external doctor and reporting the performed euthanasia to an evaluation board outside the hospital or practice.

The evaluation board will scrutinise the procedure, examining whether the protocol has been followed correctly. If not, the doctor is called to justify his course of action and can eventually be prosecuted.

Belgium

While in the Netherlands physicians called for a law on euthanasia in order to regulate an existing practice, the Belgian law resulted from a political move, under pressure of public opinion. Three medical laws were passed in Belgium in 2002: the law decriminalising euthanasia, the law on palliative care and the law on patient rights. They group legal matters about end of life, quality of care and the therapeutic alliance and are based on values of self-determination and patient autonomy in the doctor–patient relationship.

The Belgian law allows a person to introduce a request for euthanasia, which will be examined and may go ahead provided certain criteria are fulfilled. Interestingly, the 'request' element seems to have slipped, and euthanasia is widely accepted in Belgium with views along the lines of 'everyone should have a death that suits their life'. The main requirements for a valid request in Belgium are:

1   Repeated and consistent demand from a patient with full mental capacity, and under no external pressure, expressed in writing.
2   Persistent and intolerable physical and/or psychological suffering caused by an irreversible medical condition.
3   The doctor needs to duly inform the patient about their condition, life expectancy and other therapeutic options, including those offered by palliative care, and together they need to reach the conclusion that there is no other reasonable solution.
4   If the patient is not expected to die naturally within the foreseeable future, two independent colleagues must be consulted, and a moratorium of one month between the patient's written request and the administration of euthanasia must be respected.
5   If the patient so wishes, the doctor should discuss the request with significant others.

If these criteria are fulfilled, euthanasia can be carried out by a doctor after consultation with the nursing team and one independent physician. The doctor has to remain present until the patient's death, and the case has to be reported to the Belgian Federal Euthanasia Control and Evaluation Committee.

In Belgium as in the Netherlands, a second or third physician needs to be consulted about the euthanasia, but while in the Netherlands there has to be concordance, in Belgium both doctors do not have to agree, and information of and control by the authorities only happen after the euthanasia has been performed.

Every physician has the right to refuse to practice euthanasia; there is ongoing discussion as to whether, if they do, they have an obligation to refer on.

While euthanasia is relatively widely practiced in Belgium with popular support, a debate and decision in 2014 by the Belgian legislature extending the right to request euthanasia to children has caused considerable controversy. Broadening the legislation to dementia, psychiatric patients and people tired of living is being considered, causing wide debate.

What is the effect 15 years on from introducing the law?

Asking our interviewees in the Low Countries to look back over 15 years working with a law on euthanasia and how they would gauge the impact of that law, factors they considered include adverse effects of inconsistencies in the law, the risk of escalation, issues of accompaniment and pastoral care and how the law has enabled people's thinking and talking about death and dying.

Inconsistencies in the law

Several interviewees felt that the law could be improved. More particularly, it suffers inconsistencies around the interpretation of intolerable suffering, the information given to the patient and the role of the second physician.

Intolerable suffering

In Belgium in 2014–2015, 3.490 cases of euthanasia were reported. Among these 40% of the causes of 'intolerable suffering' are of a psychological nature. Patients feel that their life no longer has meaning, they fear having to suffer in the future, and they are disheartened at not being able to manage their life as they previously did and do not want to depend on others (Damas et al., 2016). For similar reasons, requests for euthanasia can also be made by people who, in the absence of any significant physical illness, consider that it is time to draw their life to a close. This was the case for 4% of the 4.337 euthanasia interventions reported in 2016–2017, while

62,5% were motivated by psychological *and* physical suffering and 33,5% by physical suffering only (De Bondt et al., 2018).

There is a very subjective element in the structure and rules for euthanasia which makes it difficult for the physician. Of course, they have the medical expertise, with which they can say when there is no more possible treatment, a criterion in the law, but in the end, they meet with protest when the patient says "this is intolerable" and "it is my right!" For an interviewee the notion of 'intolerable suffering' is one of the main problems with the existing legislation. He comments:

> Society needs certain taboos in the sense that when you open the door a little bit, someone will push it further. In the formulation of the law, the notion of 'intolerable suffering' is crucial. But who other than the patient can decide what is intolerable suffering for them? This is especially true for psychiatric patients.
>
> In some cases, euthanasia can be the lesser evil. I can understand that. But changing and turning this around from, in some cases, it is the lesser evil, to – as it is now – euthanasia is something good, and we cannot even discuss it anymore is opening the door more than ajar.

To the writers the notion of 'intolerable suffering' as a criterion in the law seems inappropriate, because the measure of suffering on behalf of a patient is impossible to assess, and what is right for one person may be wrong for another. We suggest that, if euthanasia is considered, the decisive factor should be based on a clinical decision by those qualified to make it and when they consider the patient has a very limited life span in conditions which are far from what they are accustomed to.

Role of the second physician

A palliative care physician has reservations about how the legislation regarding the role of the second physician is applied. He comments:

> There is a legal obligation that a second physician has to check if the criteria are met, but their advice has to be reported to the treating physician only, which leaves scope for interpretation. If, for instance, the second physician does not consider the patient to be terminal, how do we manage that? The law states that if the patient is not terminal, there must be at least a month gap between the request and the procedure; if the patient is terminal, there is no time obligation, and the euthanasia can be performed as soon as both advices are in. Since the advice of the second physician is not binding, and both physicians do not have to agree, the treating physician can say that he thinks that the patient is terminal and ignore the advice of the second physician.

Furthermore, while physicians have to report the euthanasia, they do not have to include the advice of the second physician. The treating physician only needs to mention the advice of the second physician. Thus, he is at liberty to say that the second physician confirmed that the patient was fulfilling all the criteria, and there is no possibility to verify whether this is correct. So, in fact, the law is very vague; everything is possible.

After performing euthanasia, the doctor has to complete two sections of a form, which serves to verify whether the act happened in accordance with the law. The Federal Control Commission corroborates 'a posteriori' whether the prescribed conditions and procedures have been complied with. They do so, examining the anonymous section of the form. If the commission considers that not all the stipulations were followed, the second section, with the doctor's name, is opened, and in the event of a two-thirds majority endorsing the decision, the case will be sent for further investigation to the Crown Prosecutor. This has happened only once in 15 years since the introduction of the law.

It seems amazing that something like that is possible, and it makes us question the process and the purpose of the legislation. While we saw in the previous chapter how evidence-based practice and binding protocols tend to shift the focus from the physician's professional 'responsibility' towards their 'liability', it appears that criteria in the law on euthanasia are not tight, and practitioners can in effect do and enforce whatever they want. If the person who performs euthanasia is the only one who has to report on it, and only after the procedure, there is no possibility to double check, and we have no idea how often they disagree with the second physician. Besides, in official records the doctor's identity is concealed in the case of euthanasia, whilst it is explicitly documented in any significant medical act, and there is no 'euthanasia' category on the death certificate; doctors have to tick 'natural death' to record it. Could this point towards some overhanging unease with the whole situation?

To the writers, the advantage of the Dutch situation – filling in the form and controlling the criteria and procedures before the light goes on green to perform euthanasia – seems reasonably obvious. There is a corollary effect of such timing which adds to the discernment of the decision making and its validity and appropriateness for all involved. Similarly, for the advice of the second physician: both reports have the same weight and should be handed in and considered in the control process, coming to an agreement between them on the advice and the line of conduct.

Information given to the patient

The Belgian law states that patients should be informed about palliative care possibilities, but there is no specification about who should give that information. Nobody will argue that a person suffering cardiac disease will turn to a cardiologist for advice. And if I have diabetes, I need an endocrinologist; if I have cancer, an oncologist. So why is there no need for a palliative care specialist to discuss a palliative care issue? Lacking such specification, the way the legislation is applied depends on the knowledge – which is not always very extensive – and communication skills of the informant.

One of the physicians we spoke to is a member of an international consortium (Poland, Germany, The Netherlands, Spain and Belgium) that examines how doctors react when a patient is asking to hasten death. They realised that doctors do not have the tools to deal with that question. They are not educated to know how to cope with that request, what to do and not to do and how to communicate and explore that question with the patient and family. Confirming the earlier-quoted chaplain's opinion, he notes:

> When the wish to hasten death occurs in the Netherlands or in Belgium, it is often considered to be a demand for euthanasia, while in fact it is not. The patient is just saying that they cannot live like this any longer. They ask for help so that their life could have more quality to it and that thus they could live it until the end. It is not always a demand to end their life. They want an improvement in their condition not necessarily an execution.

In a university hospital, they analysed 100 requests for euthanasia that came to the palliative care team; 65% of the demands were withdrawn when patient and family were given appropriate information and support and were communicated with sensibly. While a longing for it all to be over is a regular feature in patients at the end of life, a lot depends on how the physician or the team in general hear this request. Palliative care specialists are trained to pay attention to the question behind the question and explore how to meet them. People who have not learned to be comfortable in the presence of a patient's suffering may jump to a conclusion of euthanasia to steer clear of their own disquiet.

Special training in communication is provided for the palliative care team in the hospital of one of our interviewees. For instance, with the whole team of five nurses, three psychologists and one physician in training, they discussed the issue of how they listen to patients who have a chronic disease with long-term suffering and who ask to hasten their death. They examined what their answer would be and how it affects the team. They also considered how they could manage this as a team so that they were all following the same plan. The team leader comments:

> We use practical examples: we were asked that question; how did we react? And why did we do what we did? Was there another possibility?

For various reasons, palliative care specialists and teams often only become involved at the very end of the illness trajectory. If they are called upon when the euthanasia request is already mature and everybody is convinced that it is the only good option, it becomes very difficult to begin a conversation about alternative options. In order to offer real alternatives, palliative care specialists should be involved much earlier in the process.

Due care and accompaniment

One cannot underestimate the loneliness, especially of elderly people, in our society, where one person out of ten is living alone, and they are not in contact with their neighbours.

> Jules died 6 months ago in an apartment. He was living alone, and nobody was aware that he was dead. Everything was paid for automatically by the bank, and nobody noticed that his mailbox was full. There was a huge turn-over in that building, so nobody knew that Jules was living there. Nobody missed him, and he had no family. It was only when they were looking for the cause of a defect in the water supply that plumbers had to go into that apart-ment and found Jules. When they tried to retrace his whereabouts, the last sign of life was six months ago!

Such situations happen in our modern society, in which people are living alone and in which the one GP–one patient relationship as we have known it for decades is changing. Nowadays we see practices where five or six GPs are working together and a patient will see this GP today, and next week it will be another one. The doctor–patient relationship is not so close. Sometimes, the doctor on duty has to perform a euthanasia which has been discussed and prepared for by a colleague. It becomes a technical act, which the doctor on duty feels he has to accept. Because of the considerable aliena-tion in such situations, some GP practices make provisos that colleagues do not follow up on these requests in the treating doctor's absence for a short break. Euthanasia is never a medical emergency!

A GP and palliative care specialist made it very clear that if euthanasia became a 'right', he would stop performing it. It would become medically assisted suicide, which he believes would be a retrograde step. He comments:

> I am not a 'euthanastic' (i.e. defender of euthanasia), but when you do it properly it can be good care. However, I consider that there are conditions beyond the criteria stated in the law that are necessary. I even think you could make a better law than the one we have now, because filling in forms after the procedure does not help the physician to practice euthanasia properly. I can understand that some people consider it dangerous, but after many

years of practice, I think that euthanasia can be a good death also if you do it properly.

Another GP, describing herself as having great respect for life and for nature, has difficulty with euthanasia because she finds that our society cannot stand the suffering of dying anymore. She says:

> Euthanasia is very clean, but dying is not clean. Dying is terrible sometimes. It sounds terrible and it looks terrible. Sometimes it feels like our society cannot bear that anymore, that it cannot accept that there is some kind of suffering. Suffering has to be cut off. I do not agree with that.
>
> In other situations, and in my own family, I have had a different experience. The process of dying – of course we need to have pain and symptom control! – but the process of letting nature take its course can give the opportunity to start bereavement and to have important conversations. It can be healing, too, to go through the process together with the caregiver, the family and the patient. That is why I am not convinced that euthanasia is the best option.

We are touched by this valuing of life and the meaning of suffering, as it echoes our experience in our personal and our professional lives. Something can be gained through that precious time, allowing human and spiritual development for either the person or the family and the change and growth that can arise from that. Furthermore, there seems to be a learning process by which the experience of having come through suffering and remembering the fruits it yielded gives strength and hope when people are faced with further suffering.

Unlike the rest of the palliative care world, who consider that euthanasia and palliative care are irreconcilable, the Flemish Palliative Care Association promotes 'integrated palliative care', in which they consider that euthanasia can be a possible last phase of the palliative care process. In doing so they hope to guarantee that these people are offered appropriate accompaniment until the end and that euthanasia requests will be dealt with in a careful and caring way by a multidisciplinary team.

Wondering what the impact of the law on euthanasia could be on religious and pastoral care, a chaplain sat his team down. They decided they would not abandon patients who asked for euthanasia, even though euthanasia is anathema in their religions. He explains:

> We decided we would respect the conscientious decision of the patient. The first thing I say when a person asks for euthanasia is "I respect your decision, but you must also accept that I can ask questions". We don't abandon our patients. If they want to, a patient can even have the last rites minutes before being euthanised. This is our pastoral way of approaching the issue.

Stressing the importance of caring for the patient and the family, a palliative care psychologist reflects:

> The law does not stipulate that the family have to be informed, but in reality, it is very important to take the family on board. They do not have to agree, but they need to talk about it. If a patient wants euthanasia and their spouse cannot agree, they should be helped to have a conversation about it, to try and understand each other and respect each other's choices. That is something completely different from saying that the patient is autonomous, that they know what they want and they want it to happen.

To the writers it seems that autonomy, which has become a main concern, has replaced life as the fundamental value to be respected. Death, administered by the health care professional and offered as a solution, little by little replaces solidarity and creativity. As an experienced nurse in palliative care put it, the problem of euthanasia does not arise at the time of the lethal injection but in the months and years prior to that, when people experience lack of proper care and symptom control and feel isolated or a burden. The problem which our society with an ageing population needs to address is: how do we take care of the elderly and the frail? How do we value their life? What cost and resources are we willing to engage in their well-being? Failing that, euthanasia may, sadly, resemble cleansing.

A slippery slope?

Every five years, the Dutch government conducts a study evaluating the legislation and practice of euthanasia and assisted dying in the country. The third five-yearly report sees a clear increase. The total number of requests was higher, and the percentage of requests that resulted in performing the act increased from 45% in 2010 to 55% in 2015. The incidence of palliative sedation increased from 12% in 2010 to 18% in 2015 (Onwuteaka-Philipsen et al., 2017). The report recognises a need to try and understand the reason for the increase, a concern seconded by one of our Belgian interviewees, who fears a major philosophical issue is looming about the definition of what it is to be a human being:

> I have been on an ethics committee where second- and third-term abortions of viable babies which may lead to 'foeticide' were discussed. This means that they have to kill the child in the womb before the abortion; otherwise there is a chance the child will breathe and would thus have to be cared for all their life, because we cannot and will not practice 'infanticide'.
> Indications for such practices on a child of 32 to 34 weeks in the womb was an illness or handicap which made it incompatible with life; the child would

inevitably die. More recently indications for abortion in these later stages of the pregnancy are increasingly considered for a very severe though not necessarily life-threatening handicap. Where will this end?

A gynaecologist I know has stopped treating pregnant women because she was fed up with the hunt for Down syndrome and the expectations of her patients. People nowadays want one or two children, and they have to be perfect. Couples also wait till they are 34 or 35, for whatever reason, before starting a family, and when children do not come quickly enough they end up in the artificial reproductive department, and this is a business on its own.

Many people today think that they should have the right to have an advance directive in order to be killed when they don't recognise their family members anymore due to dementia. But doesn't this affect the definition of what it is to be a human being, i.e. someone who is able to acknowledge the value of their life for themselves? And then, are those who can no longer do that and those who will never be able to not entitled to all the rights that every human being should have?

This is the danger of the slippery slope: once we open up the gate of subjective decision about life and death, we end up where the definition of what it is to be human and who has the right to be a human being is seriously blurred. In the UK, too, the strict criteria drawn up for the Abortion Act have been broadened to the point that abortion is now available almost on demand, whereas it was originally perceived to be a measure to assist in very specific situations. There is a fear that a law on euthanasia might go the same way and that, for instance, people might consider it on the basis of a reflection along the lines of 'Grandmother is becoming very expensive to keep in a home, should we "remove" her?'

We remember the story of Mathilde who, considering that the cost of living in a nursing home exceeded the amount of her pension, had estimated that she could manage seven years on her savings. This is a very strange society, and one understands the shock and disbelief of Mathilde's son. The trouble is that there may be some truth in her calculation. Maybe some families start by supporting their parents but cannot maintain it, not because of a change in the warmth and friendliness of their relationship but because of what is in the bank account. Particularly with the elderly who cannot stand up for themselves and their rights, one cannot help wondering how much finance comes into it, and maybe those who say it does not may be turning a blind eye to a reality. And such gauging may happen at the macro-economic level, too, shocked as we have been to hear a director of nursing claiming that the law on euthanasia was an economical decision.

Another of our informants, a psychologist in a palliative care team, is not scared of the escalation of the demand. Patients have taught him that euthanasia can be a good thing for a small number of people, and he welcomes the fact that the law on euthanasia has brought the subject of death and dying into the open. He reflects:

> The demand has grown since the introduction of the law, but not so much as might be expected. A positive outcome, I feel, is that the law forces the medical professions, in a very direct way, to think about death and dying. Every doctor who studies at the university has to reflect on euthanasia, and they are invited to think about what they will do. This is a very good thing, because, on the whole, medical doctors tend not to talk about death and dying very much, in my experience. There is some ignorance as well as a taboo.

There are risks in legalising euthanasia, yet one also has to recognise that without a law, there will still be life ending, and another risk may be that of functioning in a grey zone where there is no control at all. As a pair of writers, we are left with more questions than answers. Respect for life and keeping people alive as long as possible, for instance, may not always be the right way to proceed, and sometimes, we may have to allow the person to die. On the other hand, actively killing somebody has always happened, but that does not make it right. It has been an important and vital foundation of our society that we do not murder or kill another person. So what are we to make of euthanasia, which, by some, has been labelled 'the final care'[2]? Maybe in a hundred years one will say 'How is it possible that the UK dragged its feet so long before they allowed assisted dying?' But it could also be that they say 'What did they do in the Low Countries? Can you imagine what happened there? They euthanised people!'

Difficult decisions

A Dutch consultant used the phrase 'sitting in the chair of God' to convey something of his experience when he has to decide sometimes to resuscitate, sometimes to do the opposite, and how that influences his attitude towards the patient. He says:

> I don't feel in control, but due to the medical and technological advances, we are making decisions about life and death. I couldn't live with the idea that I spend my professional life helping people to go on living, and then at the critical point of life's ending, leaving them on their own. End-of-life care is part of what I have to offer as a physician, and it is important to have a range of possibilities to choose from, of which euthanasia is one.

At the other end of the spectrum, we have the comment of a UK physician who, early on in his career, did not even consider that he had a choice:

> In terms of death I actually think that the first time as a doctor you have to perform an assisted death is with a termination of pregnancy. I'm pretty ashamed to say I probably did not really consider what I was doing, because I was educated to do what the patient wanted without judging. I was their servant. It never occurred to me that I had a choice. When we qualified, we signed up to medicine being all about preventing unnecessary suffering, and we should not inflict unnecessary suffering either.

Decisions in circumstances of life or death require discernment, skill and experience. They have to take account of what treatments are available and need doctors and nurses to feel confident in their choice. Established protocols, teamwork and collegial support are helpful. Ideas can be challenged and discussed, and there is more wisdom in two heads than in one. There are also patient rights, and from time to time, educated people will say they will take the decision. Sometimes there is little time to ponder. A nurse reflected on her strength and her resilience to cope when her mother died quite traumatically. She felt she managed because she had to, because her father was in the room.

> My father woke me, as Mum had accumulated a lot of secretions and was struggling to breathe. I had always been concerned that the moment might come when Mum might not have the strength to cough her airways clear. She had got herself onto the edge of the bed and banged on the table because she was struggling to breathe. I lifted her back into bed, and she died in my arms. I managed that without help, because I had to.
>
> What helped me cope was understanding that I knew she was dying. While I could have tried slapping her on the back, turning her over, at the time, I felt it would have been wrong, really traumatic and to no end. I stayed with her while nature took its course. Subsequently, I have wondered whether I did the right thing, because allowing someone to die is not the same as allowing someone to choke. However, I did what felt right at that moment.
>
> Since that happened, there has been quite a shift in resuscitation training, and the national guidance on 'do not resuscitate' has become clearer. Now, if the patient chokes or if something else happens, it must still be dealt with. That raised something very difficult for me, wondering whether possibly I made the wrong decision at the time. I have to live with that. But I may also have been right and, come what may, I might not have been able to clear my mother's airway. She was dying. It was not nice for her, but it was minutes. Neither was it nice for me nor for my father, but we had to manage and cope.

These are very difficult decisions and it has taken the nurse years before she could talk about it, but now that she can, it is helpful. More often than not, decisions need to be made on the spur of the moment, and the questions this nurse asked herself in hindsight could not be reviewed at the time. A physician had another story showing one never knows what is coming!

> I was sitting reading a book when the train slowed down to twenty miles an hour and somebody spoke on the intercom, asking whether there was a doctor in the train, and if so, could they come to the front. As no-one else was getting up, I walked to the front, and the guard there said the driver had taken ill.
>
> When I got into the cockpit there were two drivers and one of them was slumped unconscious in his chair in cardiac arrest. The other was pale and frightened, gripping the steering mechanism tightly. He explained how, when the main driver was unwell, he had taken over the controls and slowed the train down. I knew the slumped driver had no chance of recovery, because it was too long from the time it happened to the time I got to him. His pupils were widely dilated, which is a sign of irreversible brain anoxia. I decided to support the other, very scared driver. Trying to resuscitate the first driver in the tiny cabin would not be feasible. I decided my job was to talk with the second driver, helping him to stay calm until we got to the station, where he halted the train and they took off the dead man.

This doctor, too, had to make a spur-of-the-moment decision. When he walked back through the train, no-one seemed to have noticed anything. Maybe this was a confirmation of him making the right choice? Soon another pair of drivers had been found, and they continued on their journey as if nothing had happened. It had been a challenge.

Pressures, power and control

We cannot underestimate the overt or covert pressures physicians, patients and families can be exposed to in the twilight of life. People have turned to public opinion and the courts in their effort to influence decisions. In countries where euthanasia is decriminalised, the freedom of choice of professionals to act according to their personal, professional, moral or religious values to accompany a natural dying process tends to be disregarded or even penalised. Even though there is capacity, autonomy and freedom to choose for or against medical intervention, in practice, patients and physicians may not feel that free. The choices they make depend on what the patient wants, what their motivation is, what can be considered a realistic outcome of the treatment and how this can be communicated. They can also be of a more personal nature, as in the story of Belinda:

> Belinda had been dying for several weeks. She had become deaf and blind and weighed no more than 35 kilos. Her family asked the GP whether he could put her to sleep. He replied that having known her for twenty-odd years, he loved her and could not possibly do that with the intention of killing her. He went on to say that he would be willing to prepare a file for them to do it, but they could not possibly do it either.

A palliative care physician, recalling times when he experienced depression and life seemed pointless, understands very well how people become so despairing they wish to die. His attitude towards euthanasia has to do with what it means for him to be a doctor.

> When I trained as a doctor, it was a basic tenet that our role was to 'cure sometimes, relieve often, comfort always'[3]. Life was precious, a great gift, and doctors did not have the right to end it. So while I will do everything in my power to relieve symptoms and to console always, I feel I simply do not have the right to take another person's life.

In the current situation, no physician can be forced to perform euthanasia; even when there is a law, physicians have the right to refuse. However, some doctors feel that having treated a patient for 10 or 20 years, they cannot abandon them at this critical time. Feeling they have to help a suffering patient who is begging them to do something, doctors can be drawn beyond their threshold. They feel pushed to go along with the request and then afterwards pray that no other patient will make the same request in the coming months. A professional shares:

> In public, some physicians speak of their 'sense of duty' and the responsibility to conform with patients' requests to justify their performing euthanasia, but in the depths of their hearts, it can be another story. I remember a physician welling up as he admitted that some nights he woke up in a sweat, seeing the faces of the very people he had euthanised in front of him.

Whatever the legal conditions and ongoing regulations, ethical boundaries are individual. This is a challenge for physicians, who live and work in a world where shortening and prolonging life is possible and expected or accepted by the largest number. A Belgian GP said to us:

> Sometimes I think that it was easier 30 years ago. Probably it was not really, because now we are better able to control pain, and that is wonderful. But the changes in the law make us face more complex issues. A physician wrote

a book, Tired of Making Choices (Desmet & Grommen, 2005). That is the point. There are so many choices to make now. Even when you die, you have to choose how you want to do it. On the other hand, we have to follow the rules, regulations and protocols; failing that, we can receive complaints and even be sued in the courts.

It is indeed about making choices, and difficult ones at that. One of our interviewees, a chaplain in a university hospital, feels very strongly that decisions about medical intervention are the doctor's responsibility. He reflects:

> In my mind there is a big difference between physiological futility and dealing with quality of life. The law says that if a patient cannot decide, their relatives have to resolve whether they are to continue living with this quality of life. My experience is that most relatives are really not up to this kind of judgement. Moreover, they do not always agree and end up quarrelling.
>
> I try to teach our young doctors not to beg permission of the family when they decide, together with their colleagues, to drop treatment and let a patient die. The reason for that is that when they ask a family member to agree that they are going to stop treatment, six months later, this person will think incorrectly that they have made the decision by which their father, mother, spouse or child is not alive anymore. They may feel guilty, while actually, this decision is the doctor's and not theirs. So don't let the doctors beg for the family's permission! They are the physician, not just the technician, and they have to take the responsibility.

We are touched by this plea for doctors to overcome the fear of liability that might encourage them to beg the family's consent. No family member should be put in a position in which they might feel responsible for a decision over life and death over which they have no power whatsoever. There is a difference between communicating openly about the stakes and why a decision is being made and requesting the family members to agree. Understanding and agreeing are two very different concepts when family members are going through the throes of bereavement.

It has been said that people choose the suicide that suits their pathology or their life – we would like to add, if they chose suicide at all. We recall from Simon's story (*How to Die: Simon's Choice*, 2016) that when talking about assisted dying people may feel trapped in a form of blackmail. Yet the fact that euthanasia is an option can also bring peace, as in Nelly's testimony:

> When I was first diagnosed I was in complete shock, unaware that I was. After that or alongside it came the most excruciating mental pain that I had an inoperable cancer. I was a happy, working mother with three children, effectively bereaved of my future.

Had the choice of assisted dying existed, it would have been the most special comfort to me. As the shock subsided, my first instinct was to get away from a situation in which I felt trapped. I knew that I was going to die. I didn't know how, nor how long it would take. I didn't know what the symptoms were. But I knew that it was going to happen. And my first urge was to take control again.

Going through the process of scans and biopsies and meeting with the consultant, I was not in control. So the first thing I did once I got off the floor was googling Dignitas[4] to see what the options were. I reared in shock at the cost and at the bleak reality and realised I would not wish to die abroad, away from my home and my family and friends.

I had wonderful support from a hospice nurse and a counsellor, and we talked through the sense of being trapped and this fear of death and what it might be like. At first diagnosis, and even now, it is unclear how many months are left and what might happen next, and I have had the most amazing 13 months of not dying. I believe that having the option of assisted dying might help me in the final weeks to avoid suffering for myself and, above all, for my family.

Nelly's story echoes the fears and uncertainty of many. She highlights how illness brings death closer psychologically and how there can be an urge to take control again. She hopes that contemplating assisted dying in her home environment might ease that.

It seems to happen sometimes that once patients have the reassurance that if and when they need it, they can have euthanasia, they no longer want it. A Belgian chaplain tells the following story:

Bernadette had intolerable psychological suffering, and she had been requesting euthanasia for months. The moment that the third psychiatrist (for psychological suffering, the law requires three doctors to examine the situation) said that he agreed and she could have euthanasia, Bernadette said, "Well, OK. I don't want it now. I am sure that I can have it, but for the time being, I want to continue living. I will come back to you if I cannot cope anymore".

This chaplain wondered what was happening. Bernadette had asked to go through a whole request process that took months to complete, and at the end of it, when there was an agreement that she could have euthanasia, Bernadette said "No. Thank you. I will go on living". A Canadian article suggests that the very approval gives the patient a new sense of control over their situation, and they no longer feel the need to end their life (Li et al., 2017). A nurse recalled a similar attitude about stopping treatment:

Jonathan had been on renal dialysis for the last three years. He always used to say that when his time came and he could not do this, that and the other, he would just stop the dialysis. I thought he said it to provoke me. But when he was presented with the option of stopping treatment, he did not take it. When he had an infection and the consultant thought this might be the time, he wanted to carry on living.

This change of mind in people and patients, surprising though it can be, only reiterates to us the mystery of life and death and how difficult it is to come to terms with it.

No euthanasia 'on command'

The refusal to perform euthanasia 'on command' gathered consensus among our informants, and we were told a number of hospitals and hospice-at-home teams refuse referrals for euthanasia without prior discussion nor consent. Like many physicians we spoke to, they can only consider euthanasia for a patient they know and have developed a relationship with.

One of our informants told us that it happens that a GP who is not against euthanasia but does not want to perform it refers to the hospital, saying to the patient, "They will do it there for you". Unaware of the intricacies of the law or not bothering to duly inform the patient, they raise the latter's hopes that as soon as they get to the hospital they might be euthanised, which of course is not possible and causes difficult situations for the patient and their family as well as for the hospital team.

Lack of good communication can exacerbate a power imbalance and bring about collateral damage, as we see in the following story of Ted:

Sue, a widow, and Ted, a widower, were living in the same building. They had a relationship, but because of tax reasons, they lived separately and were not married. Sue became ill, and she asked for euthanasia. Her family was there, and she was euthanised. But Ted, with whom she had been in a relationship for a few years, was not warned because 'officially' he was not her husband or partner. The family were not that close to him, not even with their own mother.

That afternoon, Ted turned up at the ward with a bunch of flowers to visit Sue, and everybody vanished. The doctor did not want to talk to Ted, neither did the nurses, so they called the chaplain, who wondered what he could say.

According to the Belgian legislation, one is not allowed to say that a person was euthanised, and a patient can demand euthanasia without anybody knowing. This can leave the team in a very awkward position and can have devastating effects, as we imagine how Ted may have been shocked. Good communication requires time, skill and, above all, care and attention.

Secrecy in the context of euthanasia can undermine people's confidence in the medical profession. We heard of a woman wondering to this day whether her mother had been euthanised without her knowing, surprised as she was by the sudden death of someone who seemed so well the previous night. One understands that not all physicians can agree with this. They demand that family members are aware and informed of the request and that family members can at least respect the patient's decision. Without that, they feel it is not possible and will refuse to perform euthanasia. Some interviewees would encourage the patient to involve their family in the discussion. A physician remembers:

> Marta was a patient in the palliative care unit whose condition was still all right. Her husband was a businessman, and he had to go on a business trip for a week. The first day after he had left, Marta said she wanted to have euthanasia this week, before her husband came back. I said that I really could not do that. Legally, it was all right, but I could not do that because it did not feel right towards the husband, who really cared for Marta. She could hear my objections and lived on. She did not even have euthanasia at all in the end. Her husband came back, and there was a rapid change in her condition.

This request for euthanasia was unacceptable for this physician. What is the point of stopping the patient's suffering to start the suffering of their spouse? The law is one thing, but when you follow the law strictly, it may not be good care. Within a balanced relationship, when the person accepts that the physician needs time to see whether their suffering can be treated in any other way, and if the family is taken into account, this doctor might consider a request for euthanasia.

A young GP said she had never had a request for abortion, but if it came, she would help the person make her decision. She feels it is her responsibility as a GP to explore her patient's value systems about that act, because when they come with this question, it is really emotional, and the GP can hold a mirror to help the patient see where the question comes from. It is the same with euthanasia; the first thing is to try and find out what the question behind the question may be.

All the people we interviewed had personal criteria on top of those in the legislation when making up their mind about euthanasia. For many doctors, knowing their patient and the personal relationship they have with them is crucial in helping them assess a patient's desire to live, their (lack of) quality of life and frailty scale and the family's hopes and expectations. Hospital physicians talk to colleagues, assistants, nurses and the patient's family. For a university hospital physician, discussing the subject with students and explaining to them what he was doing affirmed his decision making.

Whatever the people and procedures involved, it is and remains a difficult decision for the doctor to make and live with. As an interviewee said:

> It does not help if colleagues tell me, "I would perform euthanasia on this person". What helps is when the patient tells me, "I know this is difficult for you, so take your time". That helps!

A physician admitted that the act of euthanasia was not a burden to him; it is very quick and takes only a couple of minutes. What is difficult is the process of decision making. This may be personal to him, and another physician's sweating might be about doing the act, doubting whether they made the right decision and because of the finality of that act. He explains:

> When a patient asks me about euthanasia, I tell them I have to think about it. It will take me one or two days to reach a conclusion, and I will talk to them on a daily basis to inform them about my process.
>
> Hugh, for instance, was a patient I did not know on the ward. A CT scan had shown pancreatic cancer. Hugh was very tired and asked whether I would do euthanasia. I said I could not. On another occasion, a doctor who does not perform euthanasia referred a person to me, having already consulted and gained consent from a second doctor, thus abiding by one of the due care criteria. Here too I refused, because this felt so manipulative.
>
> I do not perform euthanasia on command. I have a relationship with the patient and his family and make my own discernment. I want to know that the patient wants to live but that there is something in the disease that makes it impossible to continue his life.
>
> If it is at all possible to relieve the symptoms, for instance by draining abdominal fluid or by pain relief, then I will not proceed with euthanasia. Religion is important in my decision making. I weigh the pros and cons for this specific patient and try to imagine how it might be when I look back on my decision, whether I could still stand by it. I have to make up my own mind out of my own free will. That helps me bear the decision and live with it.

We are reminded here that not only do physicians have to make difficult choices, but they have to live with the decision they have made, and one cannot underestimate the burden they bear. A GP who practices euthanasia by conviction and has done so for years conceded that he can no longer do more than one a month because of the psychological burden (de Locht, 2018, p. 218). Investigating the issue, Stevens (2006) found that participating in assisted suicide or euthanasia can have a profound harmful effect on the involved physicians. They spoke of a huge burden on conscience, tangled emotions and a large psychological toll, and many describe feelings of isolation.

Decisions have ripple effects

End-of-life care comes with ethical decisions in which there is no 'good' option. Physicians and care teams have to make a judgement on what they consider the lesser evil in these particular circumstances, for this particular person, at this particular time. Hence the complexity of the decisions, as patients are usually not alone, and there will be repercussions on family, doctor, care team and many more.

A nurse said how her whole team was devastated when a patient decided to go off to Switzerland for assisted suicide. They felt they had let the patient down. She does not have the same sense of failure about palliative sedation, which would usually only happen in the last days of life and can make things much easier, including for the spouse and family watching when a patient is restless.

> Lydia was dying at home, and I needed to talk to her sons about how we were managing her care and what was in the syringe driver. I was honest, saying it was just enough to take the edge off and keep their mother settled. It was not making her sleep.

A doctor who practices euthanasia with conviction talks about the emotions he notices, imagines or avoids in the mother, the children or the spouse of patients he meets, and also in the care teams of hospitals and care homes (de Locht, 2018). People are hugely affected by the decisions taken. A UK physician had an interesting reflection on the subject:

> When a person with an incurable illness wishes to take their own life and involves those close to them in this decision, I feel we need to ask what it will be like for those left behind. For some it will be acceptable, a relief that the patient's suffering will end, and they may even advocate it to the dying person, some sensitively, some evangelically. Others, though, will take the opposite view. Suicide may have a devastating effect on those left behind with feelings of guilt – 'I should have tried harder to support him' – or anger – 'How could he leave us like that?' – or even a feeling of compulsion – 'I felt I had to help him even though I didn't want to'.

We are touched by this very sensitive plea for the impact of a decision on people around the patient. As John Donne (1959, pp. 108–109) put it:

> No man is an island, entire of itself. . .
> any man's death diminishes me,
> because I am involved in mankind.

A palliative care physician commented on the effect of the law to request euthanasia on the physicians themselves. Feeling uncomfortable, they can be tempted to reach for their comfort zone and no longer see the bigger picture. He explains:

> When we receive a euthanasia request, it does something to us. We are not comfortable with that question. Maybe the question is put to us because the patient or caregiver likes to pass it on. We cannot assume that people who are requesting euthanasia are asking for death. They may be uncomfortable with their situation and cry for help to get them out of there. We are all in a crisis, uncomfortable, and often doctors choose to treat the patient, because to offer treatment brings them back in their comfort zone. The important question to consider is how we can find ways to make everybody feel comfortable again in such situations.
>
> Sometimes people consider that since the law and the possibility of euthanasia exists, doctors have to accept that. It is extraordinary how easy it is for some family members, for some nurses, for some physicians to collude with the law. With the palliative care team, we want to check whether euthanasia is the right answer to the patient's question. That is important. Palliative care and euthanasia are not the same; 98% of our time is about palliation, about communication, about listening, about symptom relief, about bringing the family together, about connection.

This testimony reminds us how time and again, people end up talking about euthanasia while other, more important topics could be considered, such as: How can we speak about the end of life? What is the meaning of end of life? How can we live until the end? What do sick people mean for us as family members, as caregivers, as neighbours, and what can we mean to them? All these questions are crucial even when we do not know when life will end.

To go further. . .

1   What is the difference between palliative sedation and assisted dying? How would you explain to a patient and their family what might happen when the end draws near?

2   Reading through the experiences and reflections in this chapter, where do you stand with regard to euthanasia and assisted dying? What are your feelings? hopes? reservations? How might this influence your care for people who are dying?

3   In matters of life and death, decisions are not straightforward. What factors would you consider in making an ethical choice?

Acknowledgements

Text extracts from World Medical Association, *WMA Declaration on Euthanasia*, 38th World Medical General Assembly, Madrid, Copyright © 1987, reproduced with permission of the World Medical Association.

Text extracts from World Medical Association, *WMA Declaration on Euthanasia and Physician-Assisted Suicide*, 70th WMA General Assembly, Tbilisi, Georgia, Copyright © 2019, reproduced with permission of the World Medical Association.

Text extract from Donne, J., Meditation XVII. In: *Devotions Upon Emergent Occasions, Together With Death's Duel*, University of Michigan Press, Ann Arbor, Michigan, Copyright © 1959 free online access from Project Gutenberg.

Notes

1 The World Medical Association represents more than 113 medical associations worldwide.
2 A physician speaks of '*le dernier soin*' to qualify his administering euthanasia (de Locht, 2018).
3 A saying often attributed to the French surgeon Ambroise Paré.
4 Dignitas is the name of an organisation in Switzerland a number of British people turn to for assisted suicide.

References

Claessens, P., Menten, J., Schotsmans, P. & Broeckaert, B., 2011. Palliative Sedation, Not Slow Euthanasia: A Prospective, Longitudinal Study of Sedation in Flemish Palliative Care Units. *Journal of Pain and Symptom Management*, Volume 41, pp. 14–24.

Damas, F., De Bondt, W., Distelmans, W., Herremans, J., Proot, L. & Verslype, Ch., 2016. *Commission fédérale de Contrôle et d'Evaluation de l'Euthanasie, Septième rapport aux Chambres législatives, années 2014–2015*. [Online] Available at: https://organesdeconcertation.sante.belgique.be/sites/default/files/documents/7_rapport-euthanasie_2014-2015-fr.pdf [Accessed 28 June 2020].

De Bondt, W. et al., 2018. *Commission fédérale de Contrôle et d'Évaluation de l'Euthanasie Huitième rapport aux Chambres législatives années 2016–2017*. [Online] Available at: https://organesdeconcertation.sante.belgique.be/sites/default/files/documents/8_rapport-euthanasie_2016-2017-fr.pdf [Accessed 28 June 2020].

de Locht, Y., 2018. *Docteur, rendez-moi ma liberté: Euthanasie: un médecin belge témoigne*. Paris: Michel Lafon.

Desmet, M. & Grommen, R., 2005. *Moe van het moeten kiezen: Op zoek naar een spiritualiteit van de zelfbeschikking*. 4th edition. Tielt: Lannoo.

Donne, J., 1959. Meditation XVII. In: *Devotions Upon Emergent Occasions, Together With Death's Duel*. Ann Arbor, MI: University of Michigan Press, pp. 108–109.

How to Die: Simon's Choice, 2016. [Film] Directed by R. Deacon. United Kingdom: BBC.

Li, M., Watt, S., Escaf, M., Gardam, M., Heesters, A., O'Leary, G. & Rodin, G., 2017. Medical Assistance in Dying – Implementing a Hospital-Based Program in Canada. *The New England Journal of Medicine*, Volume 376 (21), pp. 2082–2088.

Onwuteaka-Philipsen, B. et al., 2017. *Derde Evaluatie Wet Toetsing Levensbeëindiging op Verzoek en Hulp bij Zelfdoding*. Den Haag: ZonMw.

Stevens, K. R., 2006. Emotional and Psychological Effects of Physician-Assisted Suicide and Euthanasia on Participating Physicians. *The Linacre Quarterly*, Volume 73 (3), pp. 203–216.

World Medical Association, 1987. *WMA Declaration on Euthanasia*. Madrid: 38th WMA General Assembly.

World Medical Association, 2019. *WMA Declaration on Euthanasia and Physician-Assisted Suicide*. Tbilisi, Georgia: 70th WMA General Assembly.

Chapter 5

Person-centred care

After considering different issues at the end of life, this final chapter is a more practical section, summarising what person-centred care can offer to make the most of the time left in the twilight of life. We look at how professionals and carers help patients move from a lower place, sometimes with simple things, and what are some of the tools and means to assist patients. Both writers are rooted in the hospice movement and are great believers in Cicely Saunders's encouragement to accompany each person on their life's journey until the end by seeking to make their life as comfortable and meaningful as possible on physical, social, psychological and spiritual levels.

In person-centred care, the intrinsic value of each person as an autonomous and unique social individual is acknowledged and respected. Ideally, the patient preserves his or her self-determination regarding place of care, treatment options and access to specialist palliative care. But who can or will safeguard that all information about treatment options, cost and consequences have been provided to and understood by the patient? In many countries there is a movement towards advance care planning to support the patient's choice and autonomy. People make a 'living will' to state what they want and what they do not want in certain situations of declining health. More generally, whether decisions involve the physician, the multiprofessional team, the patient and/or the family, when and how they are being communicated have a huge impact on people's experience.

Towards the end of life, the focus moves from quality of life in what a person still wants to achieve, experience and do before they leave this world to quality of care where the focus is on helping patients and families live with loss on so many levels and letting go of what is known and familiar. In doing so, palliative carers are companions on the journey, treading into territories which are as unknown to them as they are to the patient and the family. They walk alongside fellow human beings, frightened and bemused at the threshold of ultimate mystery.

Communication

Good communication with patients about their diagnosis and prognosis is a real challenge for doctors, which they have to face up to. With so much to research online, patients and families will soon find out if they were not given accurate information, and they will lose trust in their doctor, whilst good communication based on facts can help them appraise what they might still try to achieve in life. Austin gave the following account of the impact of honest and open communication by his physician:

> I have heart failure and was seen by the surgeon in a nationally significant heart hospital. He was very frank, saying he could operate if I wanted him to, but he would not advise it because there was an 8% chance of dying on the operating table, and in his book, that was too high. However, if I wanted to have the operation, he would have a go at it. I might be okay, but I might not be; I might die. On the other hand, if I was okay, I was certainly not going to be better than I was feeling then, because I would be suffering from the effects of the intervention.
>
> That to me was a terrific interview and I went away feeling highly comforted, perhaps because I happened to agree with him. Before we went in, my wife and I had said there would be no surgery, and I would accept the consequences. But the surgeon did not want to do it. And that was four years ago.

For many patients, not knowing is often worse than clear information, even when it is bad news. Being open with the patient and describing their situation clearly and precisely brings peace. Furthermore, discussing the care with the patient and/or the family helps them to feel they can trust you if they have any questions or concerns.

Sensitive medical communication

As soon as doctors say the word 'cancer', patients react, whether this be in disbelief, numbness, freezing, tears or shock. When this happens, doctors cannot continue providing the information regardless. They have to stop and give attention to the patient's emotions, empathise with their distress and look for the underlying worries and feelings. If they do continue, the patients' shocked state means they may still have to repeat what they have told them several times as patients in this state cannot take in the information. The following story highlights how breaking bad news can be done in a sensitive way:

> Frank had been ill for several weeks when he suddenly became much worse. The district nurse came to see Frank's wife and some relatives, and she told

them that it was possible Frank might die in the next two weeks. After that she went into Frank's bedroom, sat on his bed and said to him: "You know you are very ill". Frank said he did, and she continued to say, "The doctors think there is a strong possibility that you will die very soon".

Frank was very surprised, if not shocked. He said that he did not recognise himself being so ill. The nurse then talked with him about those feelings, and eventually Frank relaxed. On leaving she took Frank's hand and gave him a kiss on the forehead. She then left him, and he remained lying there wondering, "Why did I not recognise this? It honestly did not occur to me".

This patient was very touched and comforted by the beautiful way in which the district nurse broke the news. Having miraculously survived the two weeks, he later wanted to invite her to thank her, but the nurse would not accept. That breached her professional boundary. She was wonderfully intimate and humane in dealing with the patient's feelings, talking him through the shock of the bad news and helping him be prepared, so much so that, in Frank's experience, she became part of his circle of friends, and he wanted to invite her to thank her, but for her it was a professional contact.

Families and relatives of deceased patients report that they were helped by the open discussions, the availability of the doctor and the team, and the fact that it was always possible to make an appointment. Yet as one of our interviewees admitted, doctors are not always good with prospective and proactive communication.

In the beginning, when I started palliative care, I had to learn to be more straightforward in my communication. I was young, not that quick to talk about dying. I found it quite a difficult subject to discuss. We all knew the situation, but we were not that open to talk about it.

Families who come to the hospital are not any readier to think and talk about end of life. They come because the doctor or the consultant can DO something. A nurse reflects on how she found out that communication skills were *just as* crucial – if not more so – as the science of understanding disease pathology and associated symptom management.

Pam was a farmer's wife who was referred with quite advanced cancer of the liver. She was very symptomatic: her legs were terribly swollen, her abdomen was huge, she was jaundiced and emotionally clearly distressed. Pam looked terrified that a Macmillan nurse[1] was coming, and perhaps this confirmed for her some of her fears around her illness. She was stressed, and her tears were frequent from the onset. There was a huge amount of fear, denial and uncertainty and a clear sense of Pam not wanting to know what the flip side might be for her future.

We relaxed into very careful communication, just dipping my toe in the water, and giving some information and understanding about why her belly was big and why her legs were swollen and what we could do about that. We might not be able to make it go away, but we could do such and such to help. What mattered to Pam, what she wanted to do, was to be out across the fields with the horses. She would tell me this, welling up, and nothing mattered to her more.

Quite a lot of tears came into it, but I watched her confidence grow through this hour and a half, and then her husband, the farmer, came in. Pam and I had walked the tightrope, and she was just beginning to feel more relaxed and calm – and I think she was feeling the connection – and then her husband, with a very joyful hello, said "So what has she told you, then? Are you going to live for 50 years?" He was very jovial, but he was not where we were in terms of understanding and awareness. Things immediately escalated out of control, and Pam 'lost it' with him, and she was standing by the window banging her head against the glass.

This challenging story shows the damage of doing the wrong thing when coming into the room at that fragile time. Pam and the nurse had gone through such a delicate process, and it was very difficult and distressing for her to be faced with her husband's joviality and approach when she was trying to understand things so differently. Pam had gone from that acutely anxious and painful state to one of more comfort, reconciliation and understanding, and her husband had not. He came in thinking that the best way of coping with this was a light touch, but Pam was too brittle, too fragile, so that was quite a setback. Pam's story continues as the nurse reflects on her experience:

I do remember how well it went with Pam and her husband in the end. He came down off that bouncy place. It probably took a long time, and I knew Pam for quite a while, but it was one where I made a real difference, and she trusted me hugely.

I would visit reasonably regularly. Pam was very symptomatic, so I needed to review her care frequently. Her husband saw how much she valued my visits, how much she got from them and how she was afterwards, which then enabled him to be receptive to that as well. The relationship between them became closer. They did not have the sort of relationship that touched at a very deep level emotionally between them, but a certain honesty came out of it and a certain closeness, in their own way. Pam died in the hospice, very peacefully, and her husband was with her. He had come to a place of acceptance in the end.

Specialist nurses are ideally placed to be honest with people. They can take whatever time they need to talk about the patient's choices, their options and what different treatments might be like. They can help people understand that they do not have to do what they do not want to and that they have a say in their treatment and how they want to spend the last months of their life. One of the most valuable things professionals can do is to bring couples like Pam and her husband together and, when they cannot talk, to facilitate that. If both partners are in very different places and cope differently, professionals cannot deal with one without the other. While, ideally, everybody in the team could have such conversations, one of our medical interviewees commented:

> As a doctor, I didn't usually have enough time to address the psychological injuries people suffered in depth. If you are a consultant on a ward round with doctors and nurses in attendance you cannot spend half an hour with each patient. The ward had to function. I reached an uneasy compromise seeing some – i.e. those who needed more intense psychological support – in more depth.
>
> Doctors are now given training in communication skills, but it is still not enough. When I talk to bereaved people and the dying, they are often very grateful for the sensitivity and the medical care they have received and full of praise for their doctors. But, sadly, the opposite is also true. I've heard many stories of awful gaffes doctors have made. One client told me about his experience in an accident and emergency department to which he had brought his wife, who had advanced cancer and was in a lot of pain. Concerned to get her more comfortable, he spoke to the doctor looking after her, asking why she was in pain. The doctor, admittedly very busy, snapped back: "Of course she is, she's got bloody cancer, hasn't she".

Clearly, there is a long way to go for some doctors in developing their communication skills. Simply providing the information is not enough, and unfortunately, this is all some doctors can or wish to do. Younger doctors have a greater tendency to communicate and share decision making. However, they undergo the influence of senior doctors and 'big names' who tend not to communicate well. They could still be better educated about how to empathise and deal with the issues for patients and their families.

The following story of a GP working with a demented patient beautifully illustrates the importance of adjusting one's communication to the person one is interacting with.

> I have known Cleo for two years. She comes to see me with her husband, and we have a really good contact. One day Cleo came in saying that she was starting to forget things, and that worried her. So I took a short screening test for praxis, drawing, thinking and remembering. During the

test, I felt her resistance. When she could not think of a word, she was trying to find excuses. So I realised she might have real difficulty if things got worse.

Unfortunately, the test results were not good, and I referred her to the neurologist. Cleo's scans confirmed the diagnosis of dementia. I received the letter from the neurologist saying that he had told Cleo that she had a beginning stage of dementia and saw her in my office after that. When I asked what they had told her, she replied "Oh, there is just a little damage in my brain, nothing too bad". This made me wonder whether she had been told the truth or not or whether maybe she was told and did not want to hear it?

I told Cleo that they had confirmed the diagnosis of dementia, and then I had to be careful. This is where the spiritual dimension came into it, trying to figure out what this diagnosis meant to her and whether she worried about her future. That is as far as I have come. I have seen them once or twice since, and there is not much leeway, as Cleo is rather in denial at the moment.

In order to find the right pace and time to communicate with patients, this GP uses the traffic lights from Leget's 'ars moriendi' model (Leget, 2012). Caregivers have to feel whether the traffic light to the patient's inner space is green or red. If it is red, if patients do not want to talk about something, it is mandatory to stop. One cannot insist. If it is green, one can go on. With Cleo, the traffic light was red, and the GP had to wait until it became green. In the whole picture of the discussion, it may well be that some aspects have a red light, others a green one. Traffic lights can change in time too: a green light can become red again and vice versa.

Real communication requires empathy, trust and time, which is exactly what many doctors and families lack, and patients miss out on exploring the meaning of life and the mystery of death with their nearest and dearest.

Advance directives and advance care planning

Advance directives and advance care planning enable individuals to define goals and preferences for future medical treatment and care. They can contribute to improved communication whilst enhancing the autonomy of the patient (Radbruch et al., 2016, p. 17). Suffolk NHS introduced the so-called yellow folder (NHS West Suffolk Clinical Commissioning Group, 2013) to encourage GPs and specialist nurses to have these conversations with patients who are considered palliative. Still, there is more to advance care planning than filling in forms. A GP reflects:

> Simply filling in the forms is really not a good practice. It does not serve the patient. As a doctor you have to build a relationship with a patient. Advance

care planning is something you do several times and again and again. Some-times it is about little things and sometimes a long story. It is not about filling in the forms, yet it is important to have the choices and discussions docu-mented so as to enable a week-end doctor on duty to consult them. In neu-rological diseases, you have to grab the time for such conversations with the patient when it is still possible.

When living wills are being drawn up, they are not set in stone. People can change their mind, as we have seen in the story of Ann. After having insisted that her records mentioned that she did not want any more chemotherapy, she was now asking for the treatment, hoping it would help her see her first grandchild. An informant suggested that 40% of living wills are superseded by later feelings. A Dutch physician bears that in mind in the way he deals with advance decisions:

> People can sign a form that they would like euthanasia when they ask for it. In my book, such a document only serves to illustrate that the patient has had thoughts about end-of-life issues before. That is why it is important to have a date and the patient's signature on the document. When patients ask me about my opinion about the document, I assure them that I am willing to take their actual request into consideration when the time comes. It is important to think about end of life and that patients know they can talk about it. It is also important for their peace of mind that there is a range of choices when things are getting worse.

Rather than taking a living will or advance decision to the letter, this phy-sician takes it as the starting point for a conversation he wants to have with patient and family. Communication between doctor and patient about end-of-life care is of the utmost importance, and it cannot be merely pro-cedural or informative. It needs to be a conversation, a dialogue wherein, beyond the words, attention is given to the person's deepest needs, which are often not expressed.

End-of-life conversations

Physicians face difficult challenges in the twilight of life when they have to explain to patient and family that the end of the road draws near, that there are no more treatment options available. Discourse analytic stud-ies have identified useful communication practices which vary in how strongly they encourage patients to engage in talk about matters such as illness progression and dying (Parry, Land, & Seymour, 2014). A GP we interviewed tries to start end-of-life conversations when people become vulnerable. When someone with COPD comes home after two weeks in hospital with pneumonia, for instance, it can be a good time to talk about future options of care, asking whether they want to go back into hospital. Another opportune moment may be when a diagnosis of neurological disease is obvious and the patient is on a downward slope. He shares:

> At least once in a while the patient should have the opportunity to talk about choices: "Do you want any treatment? Intensive care?" It is important to address advance care planning early enough with neurological conditions. As a GP I need to know who to talk to when the patient cannot talk for themselves anymore. Not so much the diagnosis but the vulnerability is the trigger for me to have these conversations.

For a Belgian physician, communication about end of life seems to have improved with the law on euthanasia: people are now keener and/or more used to talking about death and dying. He reflects:

> In the hospice, I talk about end of life with patients and families on the first appointment: "You are very sick now. Are you anxious? Have you thought about what is to happen when things get worse? Do you want us to talk about that?" Some people say, "No, I am not thinking about that". We need to broach the subject in an open way so that there is an escape, because some people get very scared talking about death.
>
> To show them that we are ready to talk about it is very important, and even more that we are ready not only to talk about the technicalities of dying but also about how they want to spend the last weeks of their life. Is there any unfinished business? Who were they before they came in the unit? We give them the feeling that we are ready to talk about these things too; not only about pain and medical issues. That is very important. We have to find words and sentences by which to show that we understand and that we are human.

One of our informants, when reaching the point of asking the patient how they want to die, insists on giving in one discussion the whole range of options. He tells them about how they could die: a natural death, with palliative sedation, by euthanasia. He also discusses where they might spend their final moments, whether in hospital, at home, in a hospice or a palliative care unit. We are struck by the amount of information this physician throws at the patient and wonder whether one can expect all patients to be sufficiently aware and 'on the ball' to take it all in. It may seem that for this physician, choice is of the utmost importance. From other stories he shared with us, though, he also insisted on how he is keen on having a longer-term relationship with the patient and knowing where their priorities lie, which probably prepares them for this burning conversation about end of life.

Patients' attitudes, too, have a huge impact on how the conversation progresses. Some patients are very clear, open and ready for end-of-life conversations, so much so that they can be a support for the physician and care professional. A nurse reflected on Susanna, who died of cancer of the oesophagus:

> Susanna was very pragmatic about her situation once her disease had recurred and she was given the choice of chemotherapy or not. The consultant did not put any pressure on her at all, but she was absolutely clear that if she had only months to live, she did not want to be tied to a hospital bed. She wanted to be able to spend time with the family and at home.

Not everybody is that honest with themselves or open when it is difficult. For Eileen, end-of-life conversations wandered through metaphor:

> Eileen died three years ago. She was a wonderful lady and had green fingers. People in town came to visit her beautiful garden, and she knew the name of every flower. When Eileen was dying, her wish was to stay at home. But she could not talk about dying. This was her wish, and it was not easy, as some family members wanted to say goodbye.
>
> Two days before her death Eileen was sitting in the living room looking at her garden, and she told me, "I'm looking forward to the summer when all the flowers will be in bloom". Everybody knew she would not be here in the summer. This was her way. I'm sure Eileen must have known she was dying, but she just wouldn't talk about it, so we talked about the garden.

As we discussed in our earlier book (Proot & Yorke, 2014), metaphors are a very important feature of those delicate conversations. They are a means to reach out to the patient whilst they can take the conversation at the level they want to. They do not necessarily have to spell out the difficult words and feelings but can nonetheless communicate about them and, through them, keep the relationship going.

Facilitating attitudes

Good communication is not so much about skills as about being present and willing to engage with creativity and honesty in an encounter. The following stories highlight some attitudes which can have a profound impact on patients' and carers' experiences at this difficult time.

Listening

The best drug is a doctor's time, and the best communication is listening to the patient. Yet physicians are educated to speak and to prescribe. One of our informants, a palliative care consultant, mentioned:

> I have read that when a patient starts a conversation, it usually takes only 18 seconds before the physician is interrupting. That is the problem, because the 'doctor knows everything and knows what is best for the patient'. Every patient history has to start with listening.

Issues of power and control are often at the heart of communication between the medical care team, the patient and the family, even unknowingly. Many will have experienced a ward round where doctor and nurses speak across the bed about what is to happen without giving the patient the opportunity to respond. Research states that physicians on the ward have, on average, 4 minutes and 15 seconds for each patient and 20 seconds for their relatives, while they assessed themselves to communicate twice as long with patients and sevenfold with relatives (Becker et al., 2010; Rhoades et al., 2001). A psychologist in a university palliative care team comments:

> We are the servants of patients and families, and this is something physicians and caregivers need to be mindful of. As a professional, you are given power and influence. When I am alone for the week-end, I get to choose who of the three patients I will go and see first. That is an exercise of power: who will be helped and served first? Patients, especially those with mental illness, are not always able to communicate well and have their needs met. This can be a great disadvantage, as caregivers are tempted to attend to a 'good patient' first. Putting the fundamental question 'What do the patient and the family want? How do we know that?' at the heart of the morning patient conference can help.

Some patients or families will not accept help, care or suggestions. This can feel very unsatisfactory. An experienced nurse shared the following occurrence with a friend and neighbour:

> Carol was diagnosed with cancer of the oesophagus just before Christmas. I tried so hard to get the right support for her. One night, Carol had come out of hospital, having had a stent put in, and I phoned to see how it had gone. She was vomiting a great deal and was in so much pain. I put the phone down and went down there.
>
> Carol had not received the advice on how to manage after a stent, nor were her painkillers right for her. As a friend and neighbour, I could do a bit and give a bit of advice, but it was not my role or responsibility. I said to her husband

that they needed to request the Macmillan nurses. I couldn't phone up and do it for them, but they did not do it. Carol went to a major cancer hospital ('going to the top') for a second opinion – she challenged every finding – and subsequently died in hospital. I knew she would never make it home, because I suspected she wasn't able to accept her situation.

The PET scan[2] had shown up a hot spot in one of the pelvic bones which could have been disease spread, and I talked to her about that and explained that it probably meant they could not cure it. But she did not want to think that was so, which is why she wanted a second opinion, and she thought the local hospital was a bit second rate. It was very frustrating, and I felt a bit cross with her, because I didn't feel things needed to be so awful for her. The physical suffering could have been helped, but she just wouldn't allow people to help.

When, eventually, the Macmillan team did contact Carol, they phoned and said, "How are you?" and she replied "Fine", so still no progress was made. They said that was lovely and invited her to call them if she needed them. I just would not have let my team do that. I feel angry that Carol hadn't been seen and assessed. It was partly her doing and partly the way they operate, and things just did not work out.

We can feel the frustration in this nurse's testimony. Frustration at Carol's not letting due care in and at the care team who could have been more forceful. Frustration finally at her role as a friend and neighbour, which did not empower the use of all her knowledge and skills in this situation.

One of the assumptions that people have about hospices and palliative care is that it is a place where people are being helped to die. Keen to help, we are quick to react and clarify. However, we can achieve so much more by listening further and more deeply to what is going on and trying to respond to that. A physician reflects:

Some people have said to me, "I want it to end. Can you give me the white tablet?" Which was that person's figure of speech in terms of ending their life. My approach in such circumstances is, first of all, to gently explore what it means when they say that. What is it that has brought them to the point where they are asking for the white tablet? In doing so, something has been dissipated through engaging with their story and allowing them to have their journey and those feelings validated.

My sense is that patients who ask that question are feeling utterly powerless and frustrated about where they are at this moment, and part of me feels the same, because I cannot help them. It must be very lonely for them to be in that place. And I cannot be with them; that is where they are. I, like them, don't know what to do with my feelings except seeing some kind of parallel in our mutual frustration.

If a person says that they want to die, it must by definition mean that there is a level of distress in them that is unbearable, and the only way they can escape it, they feel, is to die. They may not even be consciously aware of this level of distress; it may be deeply buried in their unconscious, but we can assume it is there. Our instinct to survive is so profound that actually to want to countermand that instinct means that there is something very big going on, even if the patient is only aware of a few tendrils of smoke from a fire of terror deep inside them that they understandably do not want to face.

All the professionals we spoke to recognised that a wish to die came up from time to time. In palliative care such a request is seen as a cry of distress. It is listened to sympathetically, empathetically and without judgement. When euthanasia may seem an honest answer to an outwardly forthright question, a Belgian palliative care psychologist and supervisor wonders how conversations about euthanasia are conducted:

> I have reservations about the quality of conversations between patient and doctor when talking about a request for euthanasia. I fear that sometimes these conversations are too superficial, the ideas too simple. Doctors tend to emphasise the autonomy of the patient: 'the patient knows best what they want'. But psychology teaches us that that is not the case. When choosing a partner and getting married, for instance, do we really know why we want this particular person? We conjure up a whole explanation, but as months and years go by and reality pours in, we suddenly realise there are factors we were not aware of. Why should it be different at the end of life? I miss more confrontational questions in end-of-life conversations, something along the lines of: Why do they want this? What is their intention? Does the patient really know whether they want less pain and more support or their death?

Listening is crucial when people ask to make an end to their life. We cannot say that there is an easy answer, but we think that it is important to stay with the person and to show that you respect their view. It may not be your own belief – it is not our belief – but maybe that is not the point. It is about maintaining a dialogue, a relationship of understanding and support. This, we believe, is crucial.

A nurse reflects on the importance of the supportive visits of the specialist palliative care nurses, which are no longer as frequent as perhaps is ideal, and how she tries to establish an open and trusting relationship:

> I cannot emphasise enough from my experience the therapeutic value of these visits and the continuity of that support, that care and the trust built up as a result. The value of a constantly open door such as 'Is there something else you want to talk about, you are worrying about?' is enormous. It is about

being noticed and valued. And if people trust you, then they might ask you a question. I do believe you can say anything. It is how you say it.

Whenever I meet a new person, I start by trying to make a connection with them, as one human being to another, to try and make somebody relax and feel calm. In doing this, I tune in to their emotions and develop an understanding of them as an individual. It is a protective mechanism as well. One's antennae are out, because you can make things go so horribly wrong if you misjudge someone. In order to be a support, I need to understand that person and meet them where they are.

I always let the person tell me their story. I might do that through enquiring questions and comments such as "It sounds like you have had a really difficult time. Tell me what's been happening"; and then further on, "What is the most difficult thing for you at the moment?" I would then set the scene: "I am going to jot things down as we go along because I am never going to remember it all, and if there is something important we can come back to it". So you are kind of getting consent to make notes. I think also of establishing the trust in those early moments about who you will talk to, only with their permission so that hopefully, whoever it is starts to feel at ease. I believe very much in openness, honesty and trust and safety within that relationship. I think that it is important that I understand the patient's values and outlook on the world; that human connection is vital.

The therapeutic value of this sensitive and humane approach is obvious and can enable good end-of-life care. They remind us of a chaplain marking the value of connecting with patients in the day hospice, talking about their crafts or pictures or simply their friendships and life. Trust can thus be established so that, when they need to, these patients will feel comfortable to talk about their worries, questions and doubts.

Respect

A respectful, non-judging attitude can facilitate true encounter, taking us out of our comfort zone to where we did not expect. A Belgian GP never thought that she would ever practise euthanasia. Yet somehow, the way her first euthanasia came about has felt all right:

Raphael came in the practice with metastatic lung cancer. In the first conversation, he said, "When I suffer too much, I will ask for euthanasia". My colleague consented immediately, but I needed some time to think about it. I was not sure I could do it, I was not ready for that, and I was relieved that he did not deteriorate too much in the three weeks of my colleague's absence.

I saw Raphael every week. He used natural medicines, herbs and plants, which I respected. Convinced of his own truth, it was hard even to explain his pain medication to him. He suffered pain in his hip and took paracetamol, which was not enough, and refused to take steroids because he wanted his own immune system to fight the cancer.

I felt forlorn, because we are taught good pain and symptom control, and we know how to do that, but if the patient refuses, there is not much we can do. When the pain got worse I talked about morphine and saw him doubting; eventually he agreed, and we started the morphine. It remained a difficult struggle for me that I could give him good palliative care, but he would not have it. He was adamant that when he was no longer mobile and on a drip or a syringe driver, that would be the end for him and he wanted euthanasia. That was his next step, and that was really difficult for me.

Because we had that whole trajectory together and I got to know him, his convictions and his ways, I felt OK with Raphael's question when the time came. Surprisingly, when he was told I would arrange euthanasia in two or three days, he relaxed, and we had the best conversation ever. He talked about his orchard with apple trees he had planted, which yielded 800 kg of apples, and made me taste the apple juice he had made.

His apple trees gave him strength in the difficult times. His wife mentioned they were gathering photos for the funeral, enjoying the thought that his apple trees would be shown at the funeral. Both were emotional but very open and relaxed, and I wondered why we had never had such a conversation. What did I miss in the previous months? Was it my resistance to his euthanasia? I had explored his question a number of times, I tried really, but it was not until he knew it was going to happen that a whole other dimension of his life could come in the room.

As we had deeper conversations, it transpired that Raphael's mother had died in terrible pain because she thought God would forbid her to take painkillers. That made his wishes about what was to happen with him at the end of life very definite. He struggled with medication because his identity was living as close to nature as possible, and medical intervention was against this.

When I asked what gave meaning to his life at this moment in time, Raphael said nothing did, because he could not go to his apple trees anymore. Even the company of his wife and children did not mean much, because he was too tired to speak to them, and he felt a burden. There was nothing left that gave him strength or power or joy, and that gave me the peace to go along with his request to die.

Once Raphael knew that his suffering would be over in a few days, he engaged in a new and open way. Although from the start the GP had told Raphael that if she felt she could not do it, she would refer him to a colleague who could, that was not enough. The relationship was with her. Mutual respect enabled Raphael and his GP, each with their personal history and beliefs, which seemed at opposite ends, to come to a place where they could have an encounter. This experience has lowered the threshold of euthanasia for this GP, but she cannot make a general statement about her willingness to do it. She would have to see each person individually, and she could certainly not do it with somebody she does not know.

A consultant we talked to said that clarity helps him to be comfortable with medical intervention, and he wants the patient to have clarity too. Patients need to know that he does not expect they are going to die for weeks and that this is the reason why he will not do palliative sedation, which could lead to complications and a drawn-out dying process. Being clear and honest while giving time and attention shows respect. It can even make the question of euthanasia redundant:

> I manage caring for the dying by being very clear about what I do and why with the person concerned. I try to find out whether someone is very anxious or struggling and whether they would want a little bit of sedation. And then I would only give a tiny amount to take the edge off things, not to put them under or hasten the death. I think it is essential to be clear about the use of medications to alleviate symptoms, and that being the sole purpose, so there is no grey area. I feel I can do that with a clear conscience.
>
> On a rare occasion people would say that they wanted euthanasia or go to Dignitas[3]. I then saw myself representing an alternative. Usually, when they found somebody who they could connect with, feel supported by, be honest with, understand what was happening, the question of euthanasia would go, because a value came into life.

Being able to explore possible options and being related to realistically and humanely relieves the stress and helps patients discover that euthanasia is not the only way out. It might be, but in this nurse's experience, it is often kept as an option.

Honouring existing bonds

Doctors who are involved with people in the twilight of life may have known them for years. The GP may have been there at the birth of the children, at the death of Grandma and Grandpa or for vaccinations for an adventurous holiday. The oncologist may have been treating this patient for years with different lines of chemotherapy and radiotherapy, and there may even have been several years of remission with an annual check only. The nephrologist may have established a relationship of more than 25 years, seeing the patient every week for dialysis. Relationships are being made, and it is often important for doctor, patient and family to take all these steps together.

In the event of euthanasia, some doctors we spoke to would hope that they can get the family to agree to the decision. This may be a tall order, and people can feel very lonely when differences of opinion cannot be overcome.

A psychologist in the palliative care team of a university hospital explained how they involve the family:

> We start a discussion within the team about who shall perform the euthanasia and how it is for the family. In a family meeting we talk about, on the one hand, their feelings about the patient's request and how it is for them and, on the other hand, what they are worried about regarding the process.
>
> We encourage the patient to invite the family to the meeting, because it is important that they can hear it from them. It is their life, their family, and they can call their family together around them. It is about translating 'behaviour' into 'love' so they can hear it from each other.
>
> Mostly, in the course of one week, several conversations can bring them closer to each other. When there are difficulties, we may be able to help if we can work with patient and family early enough. It is very difficult when the patient is not physically able to talk and relate.

In a family meeting, some people would rather quickly say that if the patient wants euthanasia, it is all right to do it, but it is important to discuss the decision with all of them. The same psychologist told the story of Mia:

> I recall Mia, a mentally disabled daughter of one of our patients. The family was worried and wondered whether to involve Mia or not in the family meeting about her terminally ill father. They feared that she would not understand everything. When I challenged her exclusion, they trusted in my experience and ability to explain things clearly. Mia attended the meeting, and she was the one who asked the right questions at the right time!

Family meetings are a wonderful tool to ensure that all the family members are informed, that they understand what will be happening and that they can respect each other.

Autonomy does not exclude dependency

When we are not productive, our lives may be deemed to be useless to ourselves and perhaps by society, and some people want to stop such a life. Even when their physical symptoms are relieved, patients may wonder why they have to wait for their death, what is the point of their life. They have difficulty in accepting that they have to be supported by their family or caregivers. They do not like to be a burden. A palliative care physician hears it every day and challenges it:

> When patients say they do not want to be a burden, I always ask whether they have ever given care to somebody in their life. Usually they say yes. They have cared for their parents or a partner or a child that died. When asked

whether it was difficult, they would respond that it was, sometimes, but that in fact they are really satisfied that they could do it.

When I pursue by asking what makes it so difficult to accept care and to accept that they are not a burden, they refer to their children having such a difficult time in our modern society. Both parents have to work, and the grandchildren are placed in day care. For financial reasons, they cannot take leave from work. Grandparents, whether ill or not, want to be independent. They have to manage by themselves, and if they can no longer care for themselves, something has to give.

Being a burden for somebody is a problem in many of our Western communities, and patients need us to tell them that it is our job to take care of them and that they are not a burden. Not many people have given much consideration to how they will spend the last phase of their life and what sense they can make of that. Religion is out of fashion, and people are losing the sense of the spiritual. Symbols and rituals have been thrown away, but nothing replaces them, so many are looking into a void. We have to teach them again about what they can do, forgive and forget and help them consider what they should hold on to and what they could let go of.

It is our obligation to explore with the patients how they can live till the end. Palliative care is about quality of life, as long as possible, optimising it by relieving the symptoms and by giving hope and encouragement. When that fails, we have to care for quality of death. That is terminal care.

The palliative approach

Palliative care is based on the view that even in a patient's most miserable moments, sensitive care and good communication, based on trust and partnership, can improve the situation and change views that their life is worth living after all. The EAPC Ethics Taskforce stated that patients requesting a lethal injection to end their suffering by bringing on their death are a great challenge to palliative care. These people deserve the best form of medical therapy for symptom control, but also special psychosocial and spiritual counselling, based on individual respect and understanding in situations of misery and despair can make a difference at the end of life (Materstvedt, Clark, & Ellershaw, 2003).

In our view, palliative care is more than a specialty; it is a mindset, a way of thinking and looking and acting which can be applied across medical specialties and situations of care. The following stories illustrate how to develop such a palliative approach and what difference it can make to the end of life.

The whole family is the patient

The earlier story of Pam, whose farmer husband mellowed out of denial and light humour with the help of the specialist nurse to walk alongside Pam in her final journey, strikes us as a beautiful example of the whole family being the patient. We remember also the story of Peter, who died on his sofa with the children camping around him. Though not comfortable either for the patient nor for the caregivers, it meant a great deal to Peter and to the family that he could stay in the family living room and die there.

Sometimes, family life goes on by the bedside, as in listening to music, talking about what has been going on, making community and sharing the burden by taking turns sitting with the dying person. Other people can feel awkward sitting by a patient at the end of life. They may feel uncomfortable, experiencing a sort of waiting game, not knowing what is to come and when. Some may think they have or want to be there out of duty, love, care or respect for the dying person, but there is nothing they can do, and that makes it difficult. A chaplain recalls:

> Sometimes I advise people to put on the television because by the second day, the only thing they do is not talking to each other. They are not able to talk to the patient either and they are sitting there, listening to the patient's breathing and start breathing at the same pace as the dying person. After a while they may say, "I feel I am going to have a heart attack", to which I reply, "No, you are just breathing like the patient. Maybe it is better to turn on the television. You don't have to have it with noisy pop music". Sometimes I turn it on myself; perhaps we will watch a bit together. They wouldn't turn it on because they thought it disrespectful towards the patient to do that, and so someone has to show them that it is acceptable.
>
> Sometimes, families are exhausted, and we have to intervene. I have been known to say, "Maybe it is not possible for your mother or father to die when you are here. Maybe you have to go away for a few hours". Some people can wait three or four days for somebody to come before they die, but sometimes people cannot die in the company of the ones they love or for whatever reason. I don't know, I don't have any metaphysical meaning to that, but I have witnessed it.

That people seem to be waiting for someone to come or to leave before they die is a fairly common experience. Are they really waiting for people to leave? Or do they want a pause of peace and quiet? It can be incredibly tiring for patients to be surrounded by people, even if they are quite sleepy.

The following story, given to us by a hospital chaplain, is another moving example of the whole family being the patient:

> I was called to visit Max, who had received bad news that he was dying and asked for a priest to administer the last rites. I had never met Max before. When I arrived, he was lying in bed, and his wife was in the room. Max asked if I would perform the last rites. I noticed that his wife Sarah was not by the bedside. She was sitting a bit further in the corner. Max did not say much, so I thought, he wants me to give him the last rites, so I will do so.

At a certain point during the ritual, there is the prayer for forgiveness, and this is where Max stopped me, saying that he would like to ask his wife's forgiveness for all the things he had done wrong towards her in his life. Sarah got up and left . . . I thought 'What is this? What is going to happen now?' After a second, I went outside to see where Sarah was and what she was doing.

I asked her, "Sorry for interrupting, but why did you leave?" Sarah said "You must understand. It is not because Max is dying that I can forgive him. I have been cheated all my life – he has been beating me up, he has been drunk, we didn't have much food to eat, he neglected everything – and now because he is dying, I should forgive him?!"

I then said, "OK. If it is all right with you, I will go back inside and talk to your husband". I talked to Max, and we came to an understanding that he found it very important to say that he was sorry and that he was sincere, but we agreed that it would be too cheap just to expect her to say now, "Okay, you are forgiven". But Max insisted, "Ask Sarah whether she accepts that I ask for forgiveness. I understand that she cannot forgive me, but let me ask for forgiveness, because I mean it, and I am sincerely sorry".

I went outside again and explained this to Sarah. She did not say anything but she got up and returned to the room. I then continued with the ritual, and at the end, Sarah was sitting next to Max's bed, not in a very affectionate way, but she did hold his hand.

This was one of the most beautiful moments this chaplain ever witnessed. It felt like a real 'healing'. It was the first step in a process that could not be finished, because Max died two days later, but the feeling that Sarah was able even to touch him was quite amazing. Indeed, in the beginning, she was distancing herself from him and was simply doing her duty. She was there even though there was no connection or real vibes between them. The chaplain continues the story:

I saw Sarah again two months later at the remembrance service, and she told me that what happened there when he asked for forgiveness made it easier for her. The fact that at the end of Max's life there was some positive sign was important to her. Without it, she said she would not have liked to come to the remembrance service. Why would she have wanted to remember him? Sarah admitted that the day that Max had the diagnosis of terminal cancer was the happiest day of her life, because finally she knew that she was going to get rid of this guy.

Taking care of the whole couple as the patient, the chaplain enabled Sarah's healing to continue after Max's death. Nevertheless, it was very stressful for him, even after 20 years of experience. Having never met these people before and knowing that his relationship with them would end soon with the patient's death, if a mistake had been made, it could not be corrected.

One has to say the right thing at the right time, because there is not much time left to them.

Sometimes, caregivers form a very close relationship with family members. This can become difficult, because the family have to manage on their own in the end. A nurse remembers a young girl, Charm, and her mother, with whom she felt she did not manage the relationship well:

> Charm died of cancer of the cervix, and her mother came over from Zimbabwe to be with her through the final weeks of her life. A lot of my work was managing Charm's symptoms and supporting her mother Maud. I did not realise quite how much Maud valued my support and our relationship until I left that job.
>
> Some weeks after Charm's death, Maud wrote to me from Zimbabwe, but, having left that area, her letter didn't reach me until months afterwards when I was visiting the hospice where I used to work. I felt a sense of guilt that perhaps Maud had wanted to continue a relationship with me after Charm's death, and that had never been my intention. I don't feel it is for us as health professionals to do that. Eventually I did write and was able to apologise and explain I was not working in that city anymore.

Most health professionals will agree that their role is enabling patients and families to cope without encouraging a dependency. The caregiver can in no way replace the patient who has died. They try, through their professional behaviour and attitude of warmth and compassion, to help people understand that a loved one is dying and that they may have to let go of them, in such a way that, in time, they may 'spread their wings' and adjust.

Relief from pain and suffering

Good pharmacological pain and symptom control is what palliative care physicians do, usually very successfully. Key elements are to prescribe an analgesic that is strong enough to control the pain, to ensure it is given regularly, to control any side effects and, where necessary, to give medicines that are compatible with the analgesic. It is a complex and very skilled art and needs years of training. Yet there is always more to learn. A palliative care physician recalls:

> Sometimes I have looked after a patient who had been in severe pain on very high doses of opioids (morphine-like drugs) and then, unexpectedly, something unseen happens, the pain plummets and their need for opioids drops dramatically. Perhaps it might be that their psychological pain has been reduced by other means, and this lowers the physical pain, since the one interacts with the other. On occasions, though, I could find no reason why this happened.

The task of the palliative care team within the hospital and in the community is to give advice. They recommend how to improve pain medication and treat the side effects. They make doctors and nurses aware that they need to communicate with patients and that they can ask questions. Through coaching and teaching, the palliative care team is seeking to advance treatment as far as possible. A palliative care physician recorded:

> Vincent suffered very severe back pain from a cancer he had had for years. He said he just wanted to be dead. In the hospital he had been desperate because they did not know how to relieve his pain. They assumed he was addicted to the opiate he was taking, so they gave it in too small a dosage and too infrequently. One night, Vincent decided to cut his wrists. They found him, still alive, in a pool of blood in the morning. We worked on getting Vincent's pain controlled, which was not that difficult. Soon he no longer wanted to kill himself.

For Vincent, good pain control was the key. Unfortunately, too few physicians outside of palliative care are up to date and aware of how pain and symptoms can be managed and controlled. Doctors who are skilled in this art can help the patient to modulate pain medication according to their needs. Thus, for instance, the patient can be well awake for a family visit and be sleepy the rest of the day.

There are different sorts of pain, which come from different sources. Supporting people psychologically means, among other things, creating resources that they can turn to that help them feel less frightened. This might mean helping them understand better what they have been through, what they have experienced, why certain decisions were made and what is to come. Psycho-education can help with a lot of coming to terms with everything that happened, simply through sharing understanding and knowledge. Support might also mean having a room of their own, having their family there, or it may be small things like the opportunity to hear their favourite music or having photos by their bed. If people have a religious belief, they might want pictures of Christ or the Buddha to give them inner strength.

Skin contact and touch are crucial elements which doctors rarely use. They examine patients in a clinical way without realising the comforting effect their scrutiny can have if done gently. Most patients love massage, even if it is just of their hands and feet. Quite regularly, dying people, men as well as women, need to hold hands, manipulating our hands while we are having a conversation. Something of who they were in the past, inhibitions and reserve, seems to go out of the window.

Close contact with nature can be healing, too, as in Hannah's story:

> Hannah was in the depths of despair because she had very advanced breast cancer. There was a spell of good weather, so the nurses took her in her bed

outside into the garden. She lay there quietly, accompanied by one of the nurses, looking up at the blue sky and the clouds sailing slowly by. She got a bit sun-burned, so they put a parasol up for shade. A week or two later her depression had disappeared.

In our busy cities, we tend to forget the healing effect of the natural world. Being able to look out and see plants, flower beds and trees, birds at a bird feeder, the sun shining can give peace and grounding. Some hospices have dogs and cats who visit, whether the patient's own or through pets as therapy.

Healing relationships is important as well. Occasionally we have seen a person come into a hospice with their spouse, who would say "What about me? I need him to look after me!" even though they were dying. Such people found visiting very difficult, as they were still wrapped up in their own needs and found it almost impossible to expand their horizon to include their dying spouse's needs, while they felt guilty at not being able to look after them. It seems beyond belief, but it is true. There have been many family conflicts in which a dramatic healing of relationships took place, goodbyes were said and the dying person left this life at peace with themselves and their loved ones. An interviewee recounted:

> I experienced that with my father. I had had a difficult relationship with him, but during a walk he asked for forgiveness, and he truly meant it. It was accepted, and the relationship improved. Four years later he died at peace.

Spiritual pain can be difficult to address, because many people do not have a spiritual belief, and so when they develop symptoms of spiritual distress such as a loss of meaning in their lives, a feeling of deadness, a dark night of the soul or a lack of I–Thou relationships (Buber, 1937), they have nowhere to turn to to put their pain, no paradigm to fit what they are experiencing. Often their distress is interpreted as psychological pain, but antidepressants will, at most, mask a spiritual crisis. This is where a respectful compassionate and real relationship between staff and patient is a priority. From this basis, it may be possible to talk through the loss of meaning in their lives and rediscover what is important to them. We are reminded of Steven, who was helped to re-evaluate his life by the palliative care physician's relevant questions about his work and children and to find a way of supporting his bereft sons in his final days.

Some people may want to come back to a religious belief and may find the attendant rituals comforting. Rituals can be bespoke or created for the occasion:

> David desperately wanted to go home to have a last meal, drinking wine from a glass that was special to him. He was too ill to do this, so they brought

in his special glass, and David was able to have a meal in the hospice with wine poured into what might symbolically be thought of as a chalice. He was content.

A chaplain or spiritual carer needs to be comfortable talking with people of any, several or no religion. They may be the privileged confidential witness to disclosure of feelings of guilt or shame (often unfounded) around past incidents in a dying person's life which have been held secret for decades. It doesn't matter whether patients have a belief or not; they may have a deep need to unburden themselves to someone they can trust before they die. A history of sexual abuse in childhood is an obvious example.

Presence

At the twilight of life, the habitual 'doing things' mode can fall short of what is helpful or needed. Presence can be much more about entering a new dimension of being together, which can be challenging. A nurse reflects:

> The work is very spiritual as far as I am concerned. Not in terms of bringing religion into it, and I have never prayed outwardly over someone, though I have inwardly at times. I am hugely aware of the presence of God at those times and seeing His image in dying people. I think all of us can be a bit like an angel. I don't mean that in silly terms.

We can all be angels without knowing it, as Hamish became Patricia's angel:

> When the consultant said the time had come to stop the dialysis, Patricia knew her father was dying. It was her last visit to him, and her husband had given her a letter for her father. Too ill to read it, her father asked her to read it for him. This was very moving and difficult for her.
>
> Luckily there was a knock on the door, and the door opened upon a giant of a man with a long beard! Her father said, "Hello, Hamish, how lovely to see you. Could you just give us a moment?" That gave Patricia enough time to gather and refocus to finish the letter.
>
> Pat made her goodbyes and went out. She sat in the reception of the hospital having a cup of coffee, composing herself after the goodbye. Hamish appeared, and he sat with her and he did not need to say or do anything, but his influence on her was profound. He was an angel. Somehow, he helped Pat to regather what she needed in order to drive home. She thought, 'I am never going to see you again', and she never did, but she could not have driven home without him.

Angel is the Greek word for messenger. We pass on messages of hope to those we are talking to and also in how we come across, with a smile, a soft touch, simply being there. That is part of what we can do as well, just coming into a life and touching something that enables someone to endure, and off we go.

When we are not skilled enough to know what a person really needs, there can be a temptation simply to relieve their distress by giving tranquillisers, even when some patients do not want this, when they want to remain lucid. A palliative care physician recalls the story of Aung:

> Aung was a Buddhist patient who meditated continually as he approached death. At one point, he suddenly said, "Oh, I am on fire, I'm on fire". The nurses tried everything to help him, even pouring water over him to quench this seeming hallucination of fire. What we found out after he died was that there is a manifestation of the Buddha called the Fire Buddha and that Aung may well have been in that meditative state. So a literal interpretation with water didn't quite do it!

We need to be prepared to think outside the box of our habitual responses and to be as informed as possible about different spiritual states and experiences. Some conversations can be rather unusual, as with Louis:

> Louis is a gentleman who died a few days ago. A week and a half before, Louis wanted to be out in his bed in the courtyard. I went to see him, and he said to me, "I hope you are not too shocked, but I need to inform you that I actually died this morning, at 1 a.m." Then Louis asked, "Have you ever seen a dead body before?" and I said, "I have, yes".
>
> As I understood the situation, Louis was alive, but in his mind, he had arrived at a point where he could no longer tolerate the dying process, so he had psychologically made the jump. Louis was trying to work out how the people around him were going to cope. His mother, who was 90+, was due to visit that afternoon with his brother, and this was going to be very difficult for them, and they were going to need support.
>
> A most unusual conversation! It was a conversation with a man who was convinced he was dead! Sometimes colleagues try to put such a situation in a pigeonhole, saying, "The medication is doing this" and "We need to increase this or decrease that", but actually, what if it is not? What if this is a very creative way of inviting us to engage not according to what we need but according to what he wants? What if this amazing person is inviting us to think in a completely different way from what we are used to? So that actually, I know this is a bit scary, but Louis is in charge, not me, not you, not us.

This most amazing encounter with Louis and the chaplain's reflection remind us how tempted we can be to try and fit every new experience into what is familiar and what we know.

The dying person invites us out of our comfort zone, into unknown territory for them and for us – a common experience it is good to remind us of. So we can be 'the curious companion', never assuming that we share a language, a value system or even a meaning system. A chaplain comments on his position and attitude with people:

> When you Google 'spirituality' you find many meanings for the word, so which do you use? Etymologically, spirituality comes from the Latin word 'spiritus', which means breath. And so, extrapolating from that, I wonder: what is it that breathes life and meaning into this person? What is it that breathes a sense of connectedness to themselves, to the world and to others?
>
> The very patients and families we work with do not fit nicely and neatly into boxes or categories. So I walk alongside them to try and find out what they need from me or us. I want to discover what is happening for the patient. A key question that I often ask staff is: How does this person make sense of what they are going through? What is happening to them? What meaning have they constructed? Perhaps they have used that all their life, but perhaps it takes on a different flavour at this late point of their journey.
>
> Several times I have come across a patient taking my hand and saying, "Hello, Father", even though it is not on my badge. It has happened too many times to be a coincidence. I have a sense that when people draw closer to death, the veil becomes thinner and their intuition becomes sharper. Maybe there is a different level of awareness when people are approaching death; there is a sense of urgency, a need to engage with things that perhaps have been on the back burner for years?
>
> When people ask the question whether there is life after death, my sense is that this person is not asking to engage in a philosophical or intellectual discussion; neither are they looking for a theological exposition or scriptural explanation. I ask myself what the statement is behind the question or what feeling. Often it is along the lines of: "This is very scary. I am feeling frightened and disempowered by this process. I don't know how to face this. I don't know in which direction I am going". So when somebody says, "Do you believe in life after death?" I will often say something like, "You know, that sounds like a really important question. Tell me about what that means for you". I am not trying to avoid what they are saying but actually to clear a space for them to tell me what is behind the question and to explore the feeling that goes with it. In eight years, it happened only twice that somebody pushed that away and wanted a more intellectual discussion. Mostly patients needed that space cleared in order to engage and explore. Sometimes, the only thing I can give them is to witness their powerlessness. I don't have words to fit what they are journeying into.

This very moving testimony emphasises how little there is we can do. We can sometimes help people look for the positives without deadening the suffering. However, often we can only witness the incredible feelings that are involved in the dying journey: the sense of mystery and powerlessness, that letting go, that existential journey of not being able to grip onto anything, not being able to hold anything. And yet, in sharing this helplessness by simply being present in our common humanity, our help and support can be immensely powerful.

Sharing or witnessing someone's dying journey makes for a very close encounter in which intimacy holds a special place. Patients can give us so much, and we need to give them something of us, not the full story, but a little intimacy. An interviewee spelled out 'intimacy' as 'in-to-me-see', a telling metaphor for letting patients see into us. That is part of the journey. There is something about seeing the human being and wondering what they need us to notice; how they need us to be with them. Sometimes patients are not able to tell us, and we can just sit with them:

> I recall Jeff, who was just unable to speak, but the look of terror on his face spoke volumes. What Jeff was able to explain was that he had been a mercenary in Angola and that he was estranged from his family. We did not know what he saw nor what he did as a mercenary. Sometimes I asked permission to enter and sit with him. His eyes were wide open. I sat there, and it was almost painful, as if he was looking right through me, into my soul. I wanted to avert the gaze, but I couldn't, and he really was telling me something non-verbally.
>
> He held my hand, and I just looked at him. That is all he would do. Every now and then I would say something quite simple like, "Your eyes have a lot to tell", and he might nod a little. And "Your hands tell me there is something you need to connect". I took a clue from what I picked up, but I had no clue about the details of Jeff's story. But actually, whose needs would that alleviate, mine or Jeff's?
>
> What I arranged, because Jeff connected with a few people, not just me, was that people would hold hands with him and let him stare until he got off to sleep. And then, if he woke up again, it would be for somebody else to hold hands. The process of 'in-to-me-see' was completely non-verbal with Jeff, which left a part of me feeling that I was connecting and another part felt virtually powerless. All my cleverness and training did not work. What Jeff needed was not that but something much more basic. He needed my human being, core and core connecting, skin touching skin. Creating a presence for this other person and not knowing, actually having to surrender the need to know, having to surrender the desire to know.

There can be richness in our powerlessness: just being there, letting the other person see into me, not knowing what they are looking for, without trying to guide or manipulate their gaze. This too is something we can learn with experience, if and only if we can also learn to be comfortable with silence, with what may seem like emptiness, with not knowing.

With skin contact we enter into each other's intimacy. Beyond giving touch or massage, it is about being open and receptive to each other. When you do, you can almost feel the electrical charge, the hairs, the sweat, the smell, all the things you do not notice so easily, but when that is your medium of communication, that becomes very powerful. Intimacy requires a lot of respect, both to keep our distance not to overwhelm the other and to welcome them as close as they would like to come. A nurse comments:

> I am not someone who loves to embrace patients. I am very respectful of their space. But I will tune in and try and work out what that person needs. Usually I find that it isn't that they need me physically imposing myself on them, which is what it feels like to me. I think it is massively easy to make someone cry, and I would be very careful about letting people preserve their dignity.

As with the traffic lights (Leget, 2012), we need to tune in to what people are willing or needing to engage with here and now, which is not always what we think or expect.

Focus on life and relationships

Doctors and caregivers need to trust in the patient's resilience, that inner strength by which a person can adapt to new and difficult situations, redefine their goals and realise they are capable of what seemed impossible. But patients' resilience can be challenged, and they need the support from family, friends and caregivers, especially in the twilight of life. Cicely Saunders states, "the hospice movement and the specialty of palliative care that has grown out of it, reaffirms the importance of a person's life and relationships" (Saunders, 2004, p. XX). The following story told by a hospice chaplain illustrates this spirit.

> Matt had come into the hospice three and a half weeks earlier with cancer. He had already had a bi-lateral lung transplant and a liver transplant, but both operations failed. I sat with Matt and his girlfriend to talk about what really mattered to them. The story in the room appeared to associate Matt with music, as drumsticks were in evidence. Matt confirmed he was passionate about music. He had friends in the music world and acted as photographer to a group.
> One day, I was asked to see Matt as soon as possible. When we met, Matt announced that he wanted to marry his girlfriend Pippa the next day. I said, "OK, but I am not sure I have my magic wand with me today, but say what you want, and we will see what happens". Enquiries were made with the register office. Pippa went to the office to submit the necessary paperwork. The wedding took place at 4 p.m. the next day in the hospice.

Three weeks ago, Pippa was his girlfriend, then his wife and now his widow. It was all a hugely powerful experience for the family as a whole. Messages for help went out on Facebook and Twitter, and all the things requested came in immediately. After the registrar had left the hospice and had completed her job, the rabbi came in to give the couple a Jewish blessing for their marriage.

The story of loss and tragedy was interrupted. The couple had their married space, however short. Circumstances were changed. Subsequently, Matt was able to sit in the reception area; friends came in to make music, and there was talk about raising money for the hospice.

In a medicalised place, it is so easy to concentrate on medicine and illness, but this chaplain wanted to know who Matt really was as a person. Photographs and other personal items in the room provide clues which can tell us much, but the patient should be asked to elaborate on this. As a staff member, one cannot make presumptions about what the patient needs or wants or what is good or bad for them. Matt had the space and authority to tell what he needed and wanted, a vital freedom for a person on their dying journey. The patient's wishes, hopes and expectations are our guide. When the wedding was proposed, no-one knew how it would turn out, but it became of immense importance not only for the couple but for the whole family. Positives overcame dire negatives. When people realise their needs are met, they can begin to look outward towards others.

A hospice physician told us how enabling Anusha to express herself gave her a new grip on life:

Anusha, a patient originally from Afghanistan, was suffering a glioblastoma tumour. She had limited English as it was, and in addition, the tumour was pressing on the part of the brain which controls language and speech. But she discovered art. She never knew that she was good at art but produced these most amazing paintings, which completely surprised herself.

We said to her, "What do you want to do with this voice of yours? Is it something that you want to hold quietly? Is it something that you want to give expression by showing it to other people?" She grabbed at that one, so we arranged an exhibition for her in the quiet room. We also left a book and invited people to respond to what they saw.

That was one of the most powerful experiences for Anusha. She had lost her voice and found a completely different one, and people responded. Some people asked to buy a painting, others wrote what this other painting evoked for them, perhaps something very visceral, something very deep and personal for other patients but also for family members and staff. The idea was to leave the exhibition there for a week, but there was an uproar when we tried to close it, so we left it for a further week.

Anusha's two-week exhibition was hugely empowering for her. She found a voice as, without words, she was able to evoke a response from other people and hear what they were saying about her art.

Doctors and caregivers help patients not only with their medical and scientific knowledge but by giving hope, which does not necessarily mean reassuring the patient that they will get better. In the palliative approach hope comes with listening to their suffering and looking with them for the meaning of their life despite the suffering. Being a messenger of hope is helping the patient recognise that despite all that they are going through, their life still has value, that they can still give and receive love.

Hospice as a toolbox

The hospice can offer medical support, nursing support, a social work team, psychologists, counsellors, volunteers, an art therapist, a music therapist and more. The hospice has a whole variety of things on offer, but what we can never know is how people take those tools and apply them to their own journey, their own meaning process. We can only inform people 'this is the toolbox', the hospice is the toolbox. An interviewee comments on how he introduces this to new patients:

> There are a number of things that we can do to support you. You are the sculptor, you are the artist on this journey. We are able to offer you these things to help you. We are not going to force you. We are not going to tell you this is good for you, this is what you need, unless we see that you are in a lot of pain, or you might need a bit more direction, so we can ask, "Does this help?" Would that be useful? What would you think about that?

Sometimes, the hospice can help people to find words which are important for them, or find meaning by doing something, as in the following story of Mary[4], who did not know what to do with herself. A hospice chaplain recalls:

> Mary was a single lady who had given her life to her medical career and caring for her mum. Her trouble in the hospice was that she got to about a quarter to ten in the morning and then wondered: "What am I going to do all day?" Mary was not used to that. She was used to being busy, busy. The chaplain asked what she had thought she would like to be doing when taking early retirement. Mary replied that she liked to use her hands and pointed towards books about basket making on her bed.
>
> The chaplain picked up the clue and offered to get some material for her from the occupational therapy room. They brought a variety of baskets that had already the uprights, and the basket-making industry started there and then. Mary got absolutely hooked on it. She was unconsciously doing something useful and productive.

The next day Mary asked, "What happens to these baskets?" and was told the hospice sold them towards the unit's costs. There was something there about being valued. Mary was producing something, and her self-esteem went up. She was depressed, and she was coming out of it with the basket making.

It was not until she took to basket making that Mary could fill the day. It was keeping her busy and prevented her getting lost in thought, which sometimes was very negative. Anusha and Mary found identity in their creativity and productivity. Using the hospice toolbox, they ended up with something tangible of which they could be proud and which people could appreciate.

Hospice staff do not want anybody to treat the hospice as a pre-departure lounge. It is not an airport where people are waiting for their final trans-cosmic flight. Some patients dig holes in the past, and others are expecting the future, so they can lose the value of being present in the here and now. Patients live today, they live now, and to help them realise that, staff and volunteers try and find out what needs to happen, as in the stories of Ivan and Marcia.

Ivan loved to go camping with his children, but now he just couldn't do it. There is a bit of grass around the back of the hospice and we put up a tent and a BBQ, and Ivan could actually come in and out of his room to be with them. The children thought this was fantastic. They could actually be camping with their dad again.

I asked Marcia when she looked back on her life whether there is something she would love to have done but didn't. She replied, "You know, this sounds crazy: I have always wanted to wash an elephant". We got in touch with the zoo, saying we had a patient who would like to wash an elephant. They said to bring her along and that, as long as she was there before 8 a.m., she could help the zookeeper wash the elephant. She did!

These stories speak volumes about the goodwill and creativity of people who make a huge contribution to the palliative approach. Hospices are big organisations where difficult situations need to be dealt with and big decisions made. Yet full attention is given to meet all the facets of each individual patient. Meeting a difficult patient, staff wonder, 'Why are they difficult?' and then they rummage through the toolbox for what might be helpful. They strive to give people choices and guide them to see their own value whilst recognising that life is never perfect. The image of a swan comes to mind, gliding very gracefully over the water, while underneath the surface there is frantic paddling. The palliative approach is like that: frantic paddling of staff and volunteers, while patients and family usually only see the gliding.

To go further. . .

1 Encounter-presence-listening: what insights and challenges do these concepts bring to mind for you in end-of-life care?
2 Can you name three things you feel drawn to add to your toolkit in order to assist patients in the twilight of life?
3 Coming to the end of this book, what does 'a good death' mean to you, and how might that impact your work with people at the end of life?

Acknowledgements

Text extracts from Proot, C. & Yorke, M., *Life to Be Lived: Challenges and Choices for Patients and Carers in Life-threatening Illnesses*, Oxford University Press, Oxford, UK, Copyright © 2014, reproduced with permission of the Licensor through PLSclear.

Text extracts from Saunders, C., Foreword. In: *Oxford Textbook of Palliative Medicine*, 3rd edition (p. XX), Oxford University Press, Oxford, UK, Copyright © 2004, reproduced with permission of the Licensor through PLSclear.

Notes

1 Macmillan nurses are specialist palliative care nurses in the UK. Their role is second line, to advise and support the first-line nurses and GPs about specialist palliative care, i.e. symptom and pain management, as well as practicalities to enhance the patient's comfort.
2 PET scan, or positron-emission tomography scan, is a nuclear-medicine imaging technique that is used to observe metabolic processes in the body as an aid to the diagnosis of disease.
3 Dignitas is an organisation in Switzerland a number of British people turn to for assisted suicide.
4 Mary's story was published previously in our book *Life to Be Lived: Challenges and Choices for Patients and Carers in Life-Threatening Illnesses* (Proot & Yorke, 2014, p. 133).

References

Becker, G. et al., 2010. Four Minutes for a Patient, Twenty Seconds for a Relative – An Observational Study at a University Hospital. *BMC Health Services Research*, Volume 10 (94). doi: 10.1186/1472-6963-10-94.
Buber, M., 1937. *I and Thou*. New York: Charles Scribener's Sons.
Leget, C., 2012. *Ruimte om te Sterven: Een Weg voor Zieken, Naasten en Zorgverleners*. Tielt: Lannoo.
Materstvedt, L., Clark, D. & Ellershaw, J., 2003. Euthanasia and Physician-assisted Suicide: A View from the EAPC Ethics Task Force. *Palliative Medicine*, Volume 17, pp. 97–101.

NHS West Suffolk Clinical Commissioning Group, 2013. *Yellow Folders – My Care Wishes*. [Online] Available at: www.westsuffolkccg.nhs.uk/clinical-area/ clinical-workstreams-and-current-priorities/integrated-care/my-care-wishes [Accessed 2 November 2018].

Parry, R., Land, V. & Seymour, J., 2014. How to Communicate With Patients About Future Illness Progression and End of Life: A Systematic Review. *BMJ Supportive & Palliative Care*, Volume 4, pp. 331–341.

Proot, C. & Yorke, M., 2014. *Life to Be Lived: Challenges and Choices for Patients and Carers in Life-threatening Illnesses*. Oxford: Oxford University Press.

Radbruch, L., Leget, C., Bahr, P., Muller-Busch, C., Ellershaw, J., De Conno, F. & Vanden Berghe, P., 2016. Euthanasia and Physician Assisted Suicide: A White Paper from the European Association for Palliative Care on Behalf of the Board Members of the EAPC. *Palliative Medicine*, Volume 30 (2), pp. 104–116.

Rhoades, D., McFarland, K., Finch, W. & Johnson, A., 2001. Speaking and Interruptions During Primary Care Office Visits. *Family Medicine Special Series: Practice Management in the Residency Setting*, Volume 33 (7), pp. 528–532.

Saunders, C., 2004. Foreword. In: *Oxford Textbook of Palliative Medicine*, 3rd edition. Oxford: Oxford University Press.

Conclusion

Coming to the end of this book, we wish to consider whether one can equip people with ways of coping with suffering and end of life. The structure of the book around stories by which we hope to help people contemplate these difficult yet universal issues and inspire them to make their own choices is part of our answer to this difficult question. Lecturing at the end of life does not work. Storytelling about other patients sometimes helps, or one may like to give some advice if they want to hear it, and then leave it with them.

What is also very helpful is authenticity. Having the courage to be one-self, not losing ourselves in the role of the health care professional taking themselves too seriously. We need basic qualities such as energy, humour and lightheartedness together with the suffering and the living till the end. We can share stories with patients, giving the message that what they feel is normal, is human. Whatever they may feel, they are not freaks. Being anxious is not an illness, and being depressed is not a disease; it is a harsh experience. When people are about to die and have to leave everything and everyone behind or lose a loved one, it is understandable to feel sad. A large hole has been created in their lives.

Unfortunately, there are doctors who say that antidepressants are heavily underused in palliative care. When people seem to be confused, immediately they may think about terminal delirium. We feel they are missing a point. If everything becomes a symptom and people are jumping to and searching for relief or problem solving, the person may be overlooked. We have to reduce the pressure to make decisions; take time, let them reflect and look at the whole picture. Then there is a greater chance of a person-centred solution emerging.

We have heard staff say that near the end of their life, they would not wish to be cared for in the unit in which they are working, because everything seems to be considered as a symptom, and that can be an enormous moral stress. As we have noted earlier, the dying process has many dimensions: physical, psychological, social, spiritual and existential. Striking stories have highlighted that when someone starts to talk strangely, that does not nec-essarily mean that they are confused and need medication. If a patient has not eaten or drunk for some time and suddenly starts sitting up in bed and appears to be talking to someone or something not visible in the room, who are we to say that there is no one there?

Often, people are uncomfortable with the unprovable and would be much happier if a theorem was provided. Nevertheless, it is important that people can respect, if not read, the language of the dying process in all its aspects, even the more problematic ones that seem to be linked to a dimension beyond the materialistic world. Recognising the dying process means knowing something about what can happen in the last phases of life, which may include understanding about deathbed visions. It is about knowing and accepting what can happen and what can be the best way to respond to it, irrespective of one's own beliefs. It is about being able to meet a person where they are not where we think they are or should be.

How do we help people discover how to cope with all the challenges which arise at the end of life? That is a highly relevant question in a society in which people are living much longer and experience age-related disability and the questions of what it means to die for longer. People may learn by example: when they see the way well-trained caregivers work with the dying and manage to achieve something that they cannot, they may become curious. They may ask, "What happened? This man was wild and screaming, and you come in the room, and within a minute, he is all calm. How is that possible?" Then there is an opening for learning.

Maybe the very scientific way in which medicine has developed has lost something valuable. GPs who operated 50 years ago went to see their patients. They home visited, they got to know the family, they often worked on their own and a relationship frequently developed. There was less possibility to do highly invasive actions, such as transplants, and there was more care at home. Family members were naturally involved in the care – for instance, in giving injections of insulin – and so people learned firsthand that taking care is a normal part of life. Nowadays, a professional nurse has to come to the home, thus reducing the responsibility of the family. This exemplifies some of the paradox of modern care in the twilight of life: reducing the family responsibility at the same time as increasing the demands on the professionals. But in an ageing society, the professionals themselves are being reduced through difficulties of funding and organisation.

During the process of writing this book, it has been quite clear that both of us have approached this subject matter in different manners. One of us, at times, has felt tired and emotionally drained working on this subject; the other was challenged into finding a way legally to simplify these complex matters. We feel that this is reflecting the issues about the twilight of life, where every single person approaches death, whether theirs or those of their loved ones, in their own individual way.

We were curious to know about the feelings and emotions people wrestle with at the end of their and their loved one's lives and about how the medical and technological advances and their array of choices and possibilities are introduced and managed. When medicine did not know how to prolong or legally curtail a life and there were no options of more and better treatments, people did not have to wrestle with the moral, psychological, spiritual and social questions involved.

In relation to the medical care at the end of life, we have been impressed by the concern of professionals for their patients and clients. We agree that every effort to a certain level should be made to save the life of a critically ill person, but in reality, there are limits. The other side of the coin is also very important. Human beings have the right to die naturally and with dignity.

In the UK, euthanasia is illegal, and there is a widespread view that human life is of itself sacred and therefore should not be ended deliberately. However, there is much pressure today for a change to allow euthanasia or physician-assisted dying to be used in particular situations and governed by strict criteria similar to those in the Low Countries. We are touched by the notion put forward by one of our interviewees that such a change alters the understanding of what being a human is. Do we automatically have the right to do with our lives what we choose, even to end them? What of those who, for whatever reason, cannot make such a decision? Does that make them less human?

Human life is sacrosanct, precarious, precious and vital not only for the individual but also for their circle of family and friends. So when we consider a person's life or death, it is not an individual only; there is a range of others affected around them. Thus, to say that a person has a right to life or death, we talk not only of that individual but also of those affected by them and the supporters' rights to relationship, love, assistance, etc. In short, we are not islands!

In Belgium and the Netherlands there seems to be a greater sense of pragmatism and particularity about life prolonging and life shortening by medical intervention. Euthanasia becomes an option if there is no further treatment to assist the patient and pain has become intolerable. But it is still a question as to who makes the final decision to proceed: is it the patient, the family, the law or the doctor after careful and thorough discussion with the family? We feel that it should be a clinical decision based on the reality of the patient's condition, whether physical or mental. There should be discussion before the event with the patient and their family, but the decision, in our opinion, should be a professional one, taken by two or three medical colleagues who agree on the way forward, and their official report should be vetted by a control committee before the event. We recognise that this brings great responsibility and stress to the medical professionals, as they make, quite literally, life-and-death decisions which need to be handled with tenderness and patience.

Some people who oppose euthanasia also oppose palliative sedation, which they consider to be a disguised form of euthanasia. In palliative

sedation, sedative medications which may diminish the patient's consciousness are administered to imminently dying patients in order to relieve intolerable suffering when symptoms become unbearable and refractory. We are
adamant that everything should be done to control the patient's pain and
symptoms at the end of life as, indeed, all through their illness. Their comfort is a must, and the fact that lack of resources in people and time or lack
of appropriate training in pain and symptom management prevent this from
happening is deeply offensive. Euthanasia is not a problem which arises at
the time of the lethal injection. It starts months before that when patients
are left in discomfort, hopeless and helpless and start thinking there is no
future left for them in this world. Sedation can sometimes be an effective
antidote as long as it is not prolonged.

The ethical and moral issues involved have become much more significant to us since we started this project. We are inclined to say we do not
have the right to curtail someone's life, and we feel equally strongly about
whether to prolong life with excessive treatments just because they are
available is acceptable. Neither are we in favour of wishes about one's
end of life expressed in advance to be binding, as a change of view is so
common in response to changing circumstances. On the other hand, when
we consider individual issues, we can empathise with people's experiences
and are inclined to respect and even agree with the decisions taken most
of the time. We do not think, in moral terms, one can say 'never', but we
must be conscious of the patient's specialness as a person and in relationship with their family and friends and not belittle that, whatever their
background.

Who are we to (have to) decide? Who are we to judge? Probably because
of that, we feel it is a very difficult subject to regulate, and no law can ever
match every individual situation. Maybe an ethical framework within which
professionals need to be able to justify their decision making and course of
action is more respectful and stimulating of people's clinical and personal
responsibility and choices, as indeed, no regulation can be made watertight
to protect everyone who needs protection.

In addition to enhancing the sacredness of human life, we should raise the
emphasis on person-to-person training for all medical practitioners. There
should be emphasis not only on physiology but also on emotional and spiritual needs of the very ill and dying. We would also hope that it would
increase the self-understanding of the medical professional themselves.

We have been challenged and moved by the interviews and our understanding of the end-of-life issues and the way medical intervention is planned
and carried out. We are deeply grateful for the opportunities that presented
themselves in this process and the learning that springs from them, putting
some of the instinctive aversion for and anxiety around medical intervention
in the twilight of life in perspective. Finally, we are aware that our tentative
suggestions would be difficult and expensive to initiate, but we believe that

they could be vital for humanity in the long term as health and life become increasingly scientific and depersonalised.

> *How people die remains in the memories of those who live on,*
> *and for them as for the patient we need to be aware of*
> *the nature and management of terminal pain and distress.*
>
> Dame Cicely Saunders (1984, p. 472)

Acknowledgements

Text extracts from Saunders, C., Pain and impending death. In: P. Wall & R. Melzack, eds., *Textbook of pain*, Churchill, Livingstone, Copyright © 1984, reproduced with permission of the Licensor through PLSclear.

References

Saunders, C., 1984. Pain and Impending Death. In: P. Wall & R. Melzack, eds., *Textbook of Pain*. Livingstone: Churchill.

Post-script

Lessons from Covid-19

Many of the people we interviewed for this book were drawn to work in hospice and palliative care because of the personalisation of the dying process. They have a sense of privilege, being part of a team that seeks to do all they can to humanise the journey of each of the patients, ensuring as far as possible that quality of life and quality of care are sustained. And then came Covid-19, a global pandemic which generated uncertainty on personal, sanitary, social and economic levels (Koffman et al., 2020). Regular news bulletins played out the tragic and disturbing drama on a national and international level and, in health care, rapid but necessary changes to protect patients, family members and staff left everyone with a sense of unease.

At the time of writing – August 2020 – the number of deaths from Covid-19 worldwide exceeds 770.000, 179.660 of which have been recorded in Western Europe (European Centre for Disease Prevention and Control, 2020). The virus took everyone by surprise. We do not know who is vulnerable. We do not know how we can protect ourselves. Somebody in perfect health can be hit any time, and the disease progression can kill them in a number of hours.

What can these extraordinary times teach us about end-of-life care? That is the question we brought to our informants. Collating their responses, it has been difficult sometimes to separate out the microcosm of health and end-of-life care from the general impact of Covid-19 as they influence each other. It is about person-centred care in a systemic chaos and the need of systemic boundaries in order to function appropriately and satisfactorily on a person-to-person level.

Context of chaos and uncertainty

Health professionals have been caring for patients in a context of chaos and uncertainty. Nothing was known about the virus, and there was no known effective therapy. They could provide supportive and palliative care only to try and relieve symptoms and help patients feel comfortable. Lack of provision of personal protective equipment and tests was highly and para-doxically publicised. A nurse recalls:

> This was in the early days, before lockdown, and no clear guidelines had been given within our institution. Realising my colleague was sick and another had been around a Covid patient, I experienced distress. We had no protective gear. I feared for my health and that of my family, especially my husband, who suffers from asthma. I felt responsible for patients and colleagues but did not know who to turn to with my worries, as I did not want to create a panic.

This nurse experienced fear, anger and helplessness. She wanted to know and be prepared, but in those early days, there was a systemic shortage of tests and personal protective equipment. The authorities wanted to save the little that was available for the difficult times to come. There was nothing she could do except act as if patients were positive for Covid-19. She felt abandoned, having to get by as best she could.

General hospital activity was reduced to a minimum. Beds were emptied to prepare for the peak of the pandemic, which took a while to come. Stress and anxiety of staff members who wanted to be involved led to some hasty and inappropriate actions. The head of a palliative care unit noted:

> When the peak arrived, there was not much work for our mobile palliative care team. In the overall panic, health care workers focused on making patients better and did not ask for our support. However, we knew that patients were and would be dying, and people on my staff wanted to 'do' something. Frustrated and wanting to be involved, some started sending out emails and proposals. Though interesting and valuable, their suggestions were driven by hyperactivity. The rhythm of emergency is not our habitual time frame in palliative care. I needed to find ways to reassure and motivate the team and review a number of emails which might have been ill interpreted. At the end of the day, everything was useful, even the many decision trees.

Trying to deal with their own anxiety and insecurity, many health workers, including those who had retired, were drawn to offer their services. It has not always been easy to incorporate this generosity in a permanent state of emergency and ever-changing protocols and directives, which put staff resilience and institutional morale to the test (Rosenbaum, 2020a; Garret & McNolty, 2020). In an institution where one of our informants worked, 40% of the staff were on sick leave, some with Covid-19, others with anxiety, stress and burn-out. Anger at management and policymakers who had prioritised restrictions above preparedness and who were helpless to manage the crisis remains palpable amongst caregivers for whom the daily clapping, wonderful a gesture of solidarity as it was, did not match their (di)stress and exhaustion.

Changed relationships with patients and families

On Covid wards, interactions with patients were too intense or too short: patients deteriorated very quickly, and caregivers could not stay in the room for long. Protective and shielding equipment was scarce, so caregivers could not afford coming in and out of a room and changing gear all the time. Trying to juggle patients' well-being and saving equipment, they could not care the way they would have wanted to, and patients died alone. A palliative care physician remembers:

> It was all very frustrating because we were not used to work in this way and it was not in tune with our values of care. Having to say to a patient that he could not go to intensive care was very difficult. It meant a death sentence, and he was not ready for that. Fortunately, we could use our palliative care skills to relieve his symptoms. The loneliness of the patients was terrible. We missed our volunteers. It was palliative care in an emergency situation.

Physicians who did not work directly with Covid-19 patients saw patients less. Consultations were replaced by telephone appointments, and treatments were postponed when possible. Patients in hospital and people in care homes were denied their freedom. In an effort to prevent the disease spreading and to protect them, they were not allowed to leave their rooms and were deprived of the presence of their relatives. The only relationship was by phone. One could think that this is enough to communicate information and messages, but technology may isolate us more than we realise. The mystery of presence carries much more than verbal messages alone. An oncologist reflects:

> I had the feeling that I was working with prisoners. Therefore, the time I had to spend with the patients during daily visits was much longer, and conversations had to include a lot of non-medical subjects. The level of anxiety and moral pain was much higher than usual, which proves to me that caregivers and physicians are never the sole support for the patient. Even those who have no visits from family or friends usually find support in the other patients. During the pandemic, they were locked up in their rooms, alone with their anguish.

Informants working in nursing homes noted that residents were cut off from an important source of joy in their life. They could not have visitors, and activities arranged by the animation team were suspended. For some, the 'treatment' was worse than the illness. A nurse recalls:

> A lady showing early signs of dementia became so confused that she rang her children up to 60 times a day, asking them to come and fetch her because she was lost. When she was allowed out of her room and activities resumed, she found her landmarks again, and her condition eased. Other residents said, "I have had my life, it is time to make room for the young" or "If this is my life, I would rather be dying from Covid".

In the hospice too, relationships with patient and family changed dramatically. A chaplain comments:

> From a 24-hour open-door system that allowed family members to come and go or even to stay overnight where necessary, we went to zero visitors, with provision for one visitor allowed when the patient was 'near the end'. The stress on that one family member was palpable; their sense of responsibility to communicate to other family members. Patients and family members understood why this was happening, but this did not appease the distress that accompanied lack of presence, lack of touch, lack of spontaneous engagement. Staff coming in and out of patient rooms wore masks, again understood on a rational level but nonetheless becoming a block to patients engaging and seeing our faces.

We have a deep primal need, rooted in childhood, to be held, touched, stroked and rocked to soothe us. Covid-19, with its barrier gestures, has cut us off from means of communication, presence and support which are real resources in end-of-life care. It has re-emphasised how precious human contact is, particularly at the end of life.

Frustrated by the virus from delivering the human shape of care they had previously taken for granted, staff are left with a deeper appreciation of the importance of giving time and presence to patients and families. They have learned to compensate facial expression, which the patient could not see through personal protective equipment and medical masks, by varying their tone of voice, nodding and a new-found use of hands while talking. With the Covid-19 experience in mind, the relative impact of information sharing, virtual contact, physical presence and touch on people's health and well-being, quality of life and desire to live could be an interesting topic for further research.

End-of-life care

End-of-life care has completely changed in these Covid times. Caregivers could not deal with patients and families in their usual way. Everything was more acute and more complex. The whole experience was altered, and conditions were trying. Some patients died with Covid but not from Covid.

> Suffering from a glioblastoma, Maurice was unable to communicate. Unfortunately, he tested positive for Covid-19, and we were not allowed to keep him on the palliative care ward. Maurice was transferred to a Covid-ward, where he died, almost alone. His spouse could be with him for half an hour a day only.

Families did not always understand what was happening nor why. People were stressed by what they heard on the news, and families of patients who died years ago came back asking questions about the care for their relative. A physician working with elderly people on a Covid ward reflects:

> We had to discuss care planning over the phone; we could not hold family meetings nor see patient and family together to discuss their health and options of care. Dressed in personal protective equipment, communication was difficult with frail patients with hearing or cognitive difficulties or both. We could not touch.

Families suffered the loss of precious time for intimate moments with loved ones and for making memories to sustain them in bereavement. There remained a tension between their understanding and grasping logically that travels and visits had to be limited while simultaneously feeling a deep need to be at a loved one's bedside when they are most vulnerable and in need. A nurse shared how mediating between a patient and their family was beautifully poignant.

> Henry was a Covid-19 patient. On the eve of his death, I was taking care of him, dressed in full protective gear: mask, shield and blouse. When his family called, colleagues handed me an iPad to take to the patient. It was moving to see father and son saying goodbye. Henry said to me, "He is a good lad" while his son could overhear. It was very special to witness and to facilitate the connection between father and son in this special moment.

In hospice and palliative care too, work was more difficult due to all the measures. For practical reasons, part of the working week was now from home, whereas pre-Covid-19, staff were based exclusively in the hospice building. The situation has required a degree of flexibility to ensure that services could be delivered. Staff have had to learn new skills and be creative in the way services are delivered. This has at times been a challenge, but they are learning. Even so, people had to die in sometimes 'inhuman' circumstances. A palliative care physician remembers:

> Our ward is part of the hospital, and we had to follow the directives of the crisis management team. We had to measure the temperature of every incoming visitor, and only two visits per day were allowed. One day, a man whose mother was dying ran a temperature. He could not enter the ward; he had to be tested for Covid first. His mother died before the test was performed. Heartbreaking!

Policymakers were overwhelmed by the epidemic, and palliative and end-of-life care did not feature in their considerations. Lost between the reality of an illness which no one knew how to treat and diverging directives fed by what appeared to be competition between scientists, caregivers' common sense and creative efforts by the multidisciplinary team helped to build bridges. A hospice worker comments:

> We did not have a satisfactory solution for this dilemma, but providing the space for loved ones to talk and express their concern has been essential. The grand world of Zoom and Skype has also found its way into our patient's rooms, with staff doing all they can to facilitate contact between family members of patients, easing the sense of disconnection just a little. We have invested in another two iPads to allow this, although patients often arrive with their own equipment. One elderly lady had neither a smartphone nor a tablet, but by providing her with the right room, we were able to arrange for her friend to visit. Her friend sat on a chair outside of the closed window, and they were able to see one another and catch up. Another thumbs up for Covid Creativity!

Many health care professionals we talked to admitted that they took some liberty with the guidelines. They might touch a patient's arm to express solicitude and concern. When it was reasonably possible to keep far enough apart, they would take off their mask to facilitate communication and be able to reveal and notice facial expression, which can be so important in delicate end-of-life conversations. They enabled families to come in when a patient was dying for a short while and with a limited number of people. Efforts by staff to adapt and respond as well as they could to the situation, despite the circumstances, have been hugely appreciated by the families.

Triage and advance care planning

The pandemic has made us all wake up to the possibility that any of us might get ill or die at any time. Were patients fearful about seeing their doctor and being contaminated? An oncologist noted that patients he saw were more anxious about the virus they did not have than about their cancer. It was as if their anxiety took the opportunity to change target, fuelled by television and other news bulletins. A nurse was surprised at a patient's change of heart:

> Lucy had been talking about euthanasia for a very long time. That was her wish, and her family agreed. When Lucy was diagnosed with Covid-19, she rejoiced in it. But a bit later, when her health deteriorated and she felt less well, Lucy was no longer so sure that she wanted to die. In view of Lucy's declining health, we contacted her family, and they insisted that anything be done to make her better. This paradoxical situation made me query what a euthanasia request really means for a patient. Here is a person who was adamant that she wanted euthanasia, and yet when she became very ill and possibly close to the end, she suddenly no longer wanted to die.

Lucy's story reminds us of Bernadette, who grappled through a request process that took months to complete. At the end of it, when permission was cleared and she could have euthanasia, Bernadette declined. She wanted to go on living. The feeling behind both these requests may have been a need for a sense of control more than a desire to die (Li et al., 2017).

People amongst professionals and in the wider public were shocked hearing about triage decision grids based on the Clinical Frailty Scale and the associated guidelines about who to refer to hospital and intensive care. This policy felt discriminatory and was considered by some as 'ageism' or 'passive euthanasia'. Others were more at peace with the guidelines, focusing, where possible, on accompanying the dying process. Looking back, a professor in a university hospital noted that triage has been effective: intensive care units have not been overwhelmed, and the higher mortality rate in those months was primarily amongst patients with comorbidity.

Advance care planning enables individuals to define goals and preferences for future medical treatment and care. This includes helping to avoid unwanted or nonbeneficial high-intensity treatments (Khandelwal et al., 2019). During the pandemic, patients deteriorated very quickly. This required staff to think on their feet. A nurse remembers:

> At handover, we were told that Adrian had been poorly the previous night. An hour later, general alarm; Adrian was taking a turn for the worst. While part of the team was trying to resuscitate him, a nurse went to look in the patient file, which recorded that Adrian did not want to go to hospital. But if we resuscitate, Adrian will not only end up in hospital but in intensive care. Thus, in accordance with the patient's wish, resuscitation could be stopped to let the natural dying process follow its course. Unfortunately, the emergency services had already been called, and even though the patient's GP had confirmed that Adrian had given an advance directive that he did not want to go to hospital, emergency services could only stop resuscitation if they spoke to the GP in person.

This sad narrative shows how, especially in times of crisis and stress, lack of clarity about the legal status of advance directives can lead to varying interpretations with painful consequences. Some tend to act out of liability and fear of being called to court if they do not resuscitate; others feel responsible to give a voice to the patient's wish and act accordingly. Such disagreements about deep values at the heart of their work can undermine a health care team and its members.

We saw how some organisations make time as soon as people are admitted to discuss their preferences of care and advance directives. But often, patients have not really thought about these things, and many items on the form are marked 'no opinion at the moment'. Ideally, care planning is an ongoing conversation with patients and their family which starts as soon as the patient becomes vulnerable. In practice, though, it is not straightforward. A physician reflects:

> Many people in our society fear death, keep it hidden and avoid talking about end of life. In order to respect their wishes, caregivers need to know them. Therefore, conversations about their health condition, what can be done to help them and how far they are willing to go in treatment options are essential. Too often, opportunities to journey with the person are missed, which can cause unnecessary suffering.

If end-of-life conversations are started early enough, patients and caregivers are more willing to pursue them when the time comes. Care options can be talked about openly and, indeed, reconsidered. The pandemic has highlighted that proactive advance care planning can empower patients, helping their wishes and hopes to be met at the end of life; alleviate uncertainty in families and caregivers; and, when the resources are limited, guide difficult care and triage decisions with a person-centred assessment (Janwadkar & Bibler, 2020). Furthermore, taking the time to talk about death and dying and how one wants to spend the last part of their life gives the dying person and their loved ones valuable opportunity to prepare for the death, to settle unfinished business and say 'goodbye', 'I'm sorry' and 'thank you', circumstances which are known to facilitate bereavement (Curley, Broden, & Meyer, 2020).

Bereavement

Since the start of the pandemic, there seems to have been a change in personal and community attitudes to death. When deaths from Covid exceed 40.000 in the UK, the reaction to the death of an individual somehow feels markedly different, less personal, less surprising and less tragic. In normal times, people would have been able to take time to reflect on a death and on their own bereavement as friend or neighbour, but the impact of Covid deaths is somehow less than it would have been in normal times. And yet the death is of course no less tragic, no less painful to those directly bereaved because it was caused by the virus; on the contrary.

Early warnings (Constantini et al., 2020; Rosenbaum, 2020b; Wallace et al., 2020) about increased isolation and suffering and complicated grief took many guises.

> Victor arrived on the Covid ward with his wife. She did not make it. Victor lived through the bereavement of his spouse in hospital. He could not go to her funeral. This was very difficult for him, as he was denied a form of closure. We tried to allow other family members to be with his spouse for a limited time and under strict conditions, but for Victor, this was not possible.

What remained a constant for a number of patients during the pandemic is a sense of relief at being able to talk with caregivers about death and dying and about their concerns for the safety of their loved ones, whereas this can often feel more difficult to do with family members. Being with a dying person through a computer screen is difficult, and end-of-life patients may find virtual contact with families using online systems too distressing. When a patient is seriously ill or dying, twice-daily calls are recommended to family members, who need proactive information and sensitive communication (Fusi-Schmidhauser et al., 2020). Patients also broached the sadness of not being able to say goodbye in the way they would like or even the emotional pain that stems from limited choices for funeral arrangements.

In their bereavement, family members have been deprived of usual ways to honour the body, familiar rituals and the warm embrace of loved ones. Some have witnessed traumatic situations they cannot speak about or are carrying the burden of being the sole representative by the bedside. Bereaved relatives may wonder why they have survived and feel guilt or blame about possibly transmitting the disease. In a world which has become unfamiliar, and unable to turn to their usual sources of support, challenges they would have risen to in normal circumstances may become uncertain and threatening, and complicated bereavement and grief reactions are to be expected (Selman et al., 2020).

The pandemic has further highlighted the need for emotional and spiritual support to mitigate anxiety and bereavement. Patients and families were craving hope and meaning and needed to address existential suffering, feelings of guilt and reconciliation and death preparation. A palliative care lead in a hospital comments:

> The presence of our chaplain was hugely helpful for patients and staff. She did not abandon her post and remained on duty throughout the pandemic. A great thank-you to her bishop!

Unfortunately, not all chaplains and spiritual carers could remain in post. Spiritual care focuses on comfort, autonomy, meaningfulness, preparedness and interpersonal connection. While chaplains play a crucial role in this, skilled listening with kindness and compassion and an intrinsic unconditional acceptance and recognition of human worth can be provided by all staff members (Proulx & Jacelon, 2004; Yuichi Clark, Joseph, & Humpfreys, 2019).

Caregiver (di)stress and support

Like so many, we have been moved by the caregivers who worked on the front line in extremely difficult circumstances. Fear for their own health and safety was pervasive. On the Covid ward of which an informant was in charge, 90% of the staff were contaminated, and the team suffered the loss of one of them, a nurse who died from being infected while doing her job. A hospice chaplain remembers:

> For staff, fear was an understandable undercurrent. The Covid status of patients coming in from hospital was unknown. The tension between reasonable self-protection and the drive to sustain a safe, compassionate, caring and personalised experience of care was very real. Doing what was undoubtedly an emotionally as well as physically draining job, the sense of solidarity amongst staff was evident, as was the humour that acted as an occasional pressure valve.

Caregivers were frustrated by their inability to work the way they knew how to do their job well: they could not offer proper accompaniment, they were at a loss realising how the bodies were disposed of, and they could not attend funerals of people they had known, some for several years. Caregivers are at risk of moral injury resulting from those personal or ethical conflicts and of secondary or vicarious trauma triggered by repeated empathic engagement with sadness and loss (Selman et al., 2020).

The overall number and manner of deaths took their toll too. In a university hospital, 1 in 2 of the patients over the age of 70 they cared for died. Fear for the devastation of breathlessness and patients dying from choking was pounding. Aware that severe shortness of breath in patients can be highly distressing, GPs in nursing and care homes were tempted to prescribe high levels of sedation to protect the staff from having to witness it.

An informant working in palliative care recognised that being used to work in a team and to deal with moral distress, suffering and dying, he felt better prepared than other health professionals:

> 'Soft' skills of palliative care are so necessary in a crisis like this. Proper communication, proper pain and symptom control, dealing with the suffering of

patients and their families are essential in our health system. Still, this strange time has confirmed how devastating breathlessness is as a symptom, and I am concerned about what happened in the field and what impact it may have on the caregivers.

For all our informants, this pandemic has heightened their awareness that health care workers across disciplines need to be better prepared to prevent, relieve and deal with pain and suffering in patients and families, and several voices have drawn attention to what palliative care has to offer to build capacity in these matters across disciplines and specialties (Rosa et al., 2020; Radbruch et al., 2020).

An informant noted that, unfortunately, her specialty was not represented in the crisis management team of the hospital. The team composed of consultants in pneumology, resuscitation, geriatrics, infectious diseases and intensive care reflected the earlier noted focus on emergency and getting patients better. When an ethics committee was set up, this palliative care consultant had been invited and was able to contribute and share their expertise. They discussed criteria for triage, palliative and supportive therapies and how to manage end-of-life distress. They also talked about how to organise family visits, psychological support of families and caregivers and bereavement rituals in an emergency situation.

Boundaries and self-care

The Covid-19 experience has required a re-appraisal of professional boundaries but not to the detriment of self-care. Health care workers need to take care of themselves in order to care well for the sick and the dying. Self-care is crucial. A hospice chaplain reflects:

> In terms of self-care, being with patients has reminded me of how precious time and relationships are. Connecting with family and friends has become a priority. Taking time to rest, to notice and look after my body, has become as important as clearing space for prayer and reflection.

Clinicians are trained to put aside their own feelings and to focus on patient well-being and care first. This may be why informants struggled to understand and respond to our question about self-care and boundaries. Even more so as the concept of self-care may feel at odds with a plea to outstrip personal limits and ignore boundaries in times of crisis.

For some of our informants, what has been helpful was simply being there, with all the others. They have experienced a great sense of solidarity in the team, each playing their part, checking regularly with each other how they were doing and more generally supporting each other. Supervision, maintained through Skype, helped to put words to experiences, hold emotions and recognise that they were not alone in what they experienced.

Self-care relies on self-awareness along with resilience and social support. Being able to take breaks and disconnect from the event, feeling prepared and supported in their role, being aware or informed of available resources and services and adequate supervision and peer support are particularly recommended for self-care in health care emergencies (Wallace et al., 2020; Radbruch et al., 2020).

Talking with people with similar experiences is precious and is ongoing for our informants. After the peak of the pandemic, it has helped them in acknowledging their enduring anxiety, attention deficit, fatigue and other post-traumatic stress symptoms and in recognising their fear of it all starting again. In some institutions, staff were helped by good leadership and synergy between management, ministry and caregivers. Unfortunately, for others, weaknesses in the organisation or tension in the team were exposed in this stressful time, which added to the burden on staff and affected what happened to the patients.

Conclusion

The pandemic has demonstrated our fragility and shattered the illusion that we control our lives. It has laid bare the vulnerability of the Western cultural and political model of individualism and continuing economic growth. It has posed the ethical question of the place of the elderly and the frail in a society based on performance and productivity, revealing a reality that was hidden. This event has been deeply traumatic not just for those directly affected by the virus but for all of us, and it may have a knock-on effect for many years to come in terms of delayed traumatic reactions needing psychological support. Already we can see people going into dissociation and denial, crowding onto the beaches, pretending: 'I'm tough, I don't need a mask'.

What is most positive on micro and macro levels is the heart-warming mobilisation of solidarity amongst front-line workers and the wider public. People cooked meals and sewed equipment for health workers or, more generally, shopped for and talked to neighbours they had not met before. The pandemic has demonstrated the importance of cooperation rather than competition in the way we live and work.

In end-of-life care, Covid-19 has reinforced how centrally important the family is in supporting a patient and how traumatic it can be for bereavement when the dying person and their family cannot say goodbye. It has revealed the need for increased capacity for clinicians and caregivers, across disciplines and specialties, in pain and symptom control, advance care planning and end-of-life conversations (Rosa et al., 2020). It has exposed the central importance of self-care and support for the health workers and of person-centred assessment and decision-making when rationing care (Fadul, Elsayem, & Bruera, 2020; Hanson, 2020).

Despite and because of the lessons learnt, we hope that we may soon come through the Covid-19 pandemic and return to a time when death is anticipated, experienced and recalled as it should be; that we may be able once again to share in the collective experience and grief sharing of normal funerals and to offer whatever comfort and love we can to the dying and to the bereaved. As for the caregivers, the motto could be 'together we go further' – or, as one of our interviewees said, *"My humanity as a caregiver is safeguarded by not being alone".*

References

Constantini, M., Sleeman, K. E., Peruselli, C. & Higginson, I., 2020. Response and Role of Palliative Care During the Covid-19 Pandemic: A National Telephone Survey of Hospices in Italy. *Palliative Medicine*, Volume published online. doi: 10.1177/0269216320920780.

Curley, M. A., Broden, E. G. & Meyer, E. C., 2020. Alone, the Hardest Part. *Intensive Care Medicine*, Volume published online. doi: 10.1007/s00134-020-06145-9.

European Centre for Disease Prevention and Control, 2020. *Covid-19*. [Online] Available at: https://qap.ecdc.europa.eu/public/extensions/COVID-19/COVID-19.html [Accessed 17 August 2020].

Fadul, N., Elsayem, E. A. & Bruera, E., 2020. Integration of Palliative Care Into COVID-19 Pandemic Planning. *BMJ Supportive & Palliative Care*, Epub ahead of print (12/8/20), pp. 1–5. doi: 10.1136/ bmjspcare-2020-002364.

Fusi-Schmidhauser, T., Preston, N. J., Keller, N. & Gamondi, C., 2020. Conservative Management of COVID-19 Patients – Emergency Palliative Care in Action. *Journal of Pain and Symptom Management*, Volume 60 (1), pp. e27-e30. doi: 10.1016/j.jpainsymman.2020.03.030.

Garret, J. R. & McNolty, L. A., 2020. More Than Warm Fuzzy Feelings: The Imperative of Institutional Morale in Hospital Pandemic Responses. *The American Journal of Bioethics*, Volume 20 (7), pp. 92–94. doi: 10.1080/15265161.2020.1779407.

Hanson, L. C., 2020. We Will All Be Changed: Palliative Care Transformation in the Time of COVID-19. *Journal of Palliative Medicine*, Volume published online. doi: 10.1089/jpm.2020.0446.

Janwadkar, A. S. & Bibler, T. M., 2020. Ethical Challenges in Advance Care Planning During the COVID-19 Pandemic. *The American Journal of Bioethics*, Volume 20 (7), pp. 202–204.

Khandelwal, N. et al., 2019. Pragmatic Methods to Avoid Intensive Care Unit Admission When It Does Not Align With Patient and Family Goals. *The Lancet Respiratory Medicine*, July, Volume 7 (7), pp. 613–625.

Koffman, J., Gross, J., Etkind, S. N. & Selman, L., 2020. Uncertainty and COVID-19: How Are We To Respond? *Journal of the Royal Society of Medicine*, Volume 113 (6), pp. 211–216. doi: 10.1177/0141076820930665.

Li, M., Watt, S., Escaf, M., Gardam, M., Heesters, A., O'Leary, G. & Rodin, G., 2017. Medical Assistance in Dying – Implementing a Hospital-Based Program in Canada. *The New England Journal of Medicine*, Volume 376 (21), pp. 2082–2088.

Proulx, K. & Jacelon, C., 2004. Dying With Dignity: The Good Patient Versus the Good Death. *American Journal of Hospice and Palliative Medicine*, Volume 21, pp. 116–120.

Radbruch, L., Knaul, F. M., de Lima, L., de Joncheere, C. & Bhadelia, A., 2020. The Key Role of Palliative Care in Response to the COVID-19 Tsunami of Suffering. *The Lancet*, Volume 395 (10235), pp. 1467–1469.

Rosa, W. E. et al., 2020. Coronavirus Disease 2019 as an Opportunity to Move Toward Transdisciplinary Palliative Care. *Journal of Palliative Medicine*. doi: 10.1089/jpm.2020.0306.

Rosenbaum, L., 2020a. Facing COVID-19 in Italy – Ethics, Logistics, and Therapeutics on the Epidemic's Front Line. *The New England Journal of Medicine*, Volume published online. doi: 10.1056/NEJMp2005492.

Rosenbaum, L., 2020b. Harnessing our humanity – how Washington's health care workers have risen to the pandemic challenge. *The New England Journal of Medicine*, Volume 382 (22), pp. 2069–2071. doi: 10.1056/NEJMp2007466.

Selman, L. E. et al., 2020. Bereavement Support on the Frontline of COVID-19: Recommendations for Hospital Clinicians. *Journal of Pain and Symptom Management*, Volume 60 (2), pp. e81-e86. doi: 10.1016/j.jpainsymman.2020.04.024.

Wallace, C. L., Wladkowski, S. P., Gibson, A. & White, P., 2020. Grief During the COVID-19 Pandemic: Considerations for Palliative Care Providers. *Journal of Pain and Symptom Management*, Volume 60 (1), pp. e70-e76.

Yuichi Clark, P., Joseph, D. M. & Humpfreys, J., 2019. Cultural, Psychological, and Spiritual Dimensions of Palliative Care in Humanitarian Crises. In: E. Waldman & M. Glass, eds., *A Field Manual for Palliative Care in Humanitarian Crises*. Oxford: Oxford University Press, pp. 127–132.

Glossary

Assisted dying Helping someone to die by pointing them in the direction of a website through which they can find the necessary products or of an address, in Switzerland for instance, where they can be helped to die.

Assisted suicide A practice that is legal in Switzerland under certain conditions in which someone prepares a lethal cocktail, which the patient has to administer himself, usually by drinking.

Bile duct cancer or cholangiocarcinoma Cancer that originates in the bile ducts which drain bile from the liver into the small intestine. No potentially curative treatment exists except surgery, but most people have advanced-stage disease at presentation and are inoperable at the time of diagnosis.

COPD or chronic obstructive pulmonary disease A progressive lung disease characterised by breathing problems and poor air flow.

CT scan or computerised axial tomography scan A medical imaging technology that produces cross-sectional representations of the body using X-rays and a computer.

DNAR or do not attempt resuscitation Decision made by a patient and which is noted in their file that, in case of an event, they do not want paramedics or doctors to make further efforts to prolong their life.

Euthanasia Medical intervention to end a person's life. Doctor and patient have to set a time for administering a syringe that will kill the patient in a matter of minutes.

Glioblastoma An aggressive type of cancer that can occur in the brain or spinal cord.

ICU or intensive care unit Hospital ward for patients with severe and life-threatening illnesses and injuries, which require constant, close monitoring and specialist equipment to ensure normal bodily functions.

IPA or interpretative phenomenological analysis A qualitative research methodology concerned with trying to understand lived experience and the meanings which those experiences hold for the participants.

Macmillan nurse Specialist palliative care nurse in the UK. Their role is to advise and support about symptom and pain management as well as practicalities which can enhance the patient's comfort.

MND or motor neurone disease A neurodegenerative disorder consisting in a progressive weakening of all the muscles in the body, which eventually affects the ability to breathe and causes death.

Pancreatectomy Surgery to remove the pancreas.

PET scan or positron-emission tomography scan A nuclear medicine functional imaging technique that is used to observe metabolic processes in the body as an aid to the diagnosis of disease.

Physician-assisted dying An alternative expression for euthanasia which clarifies that it is a doctor who administers the lethal drug to the patient.

PTSD or post-traumatic stress disorder A mental health condition that can occur after experiencing or witnessing a terrifying event. Symptoms may include flashbacks, nightmares, severe anxiety, uncontrollable thoughts about the event and dissociation.

Reanastomosis Surgery by which after part of the gut (or blood vessel) has been removed, the divided gut (or vessel) is reunited.

Sedation (or palliative sedation) A medical intervention by which sedative medications which may diminish the patient's consciousness are administered (to imminently dying patients) to relieve intolerable suffering when symptoms become unbearable and refractory.

SPICT Supportive and Palliative Care Indicators Tool.

WHOQOL The World Health Organization Quality of Life Instruments

Index

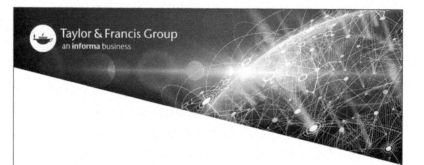